TABLE of CONTENTS

Anatomy and Pathology: The World's Best Anatomical Charts

T0199955

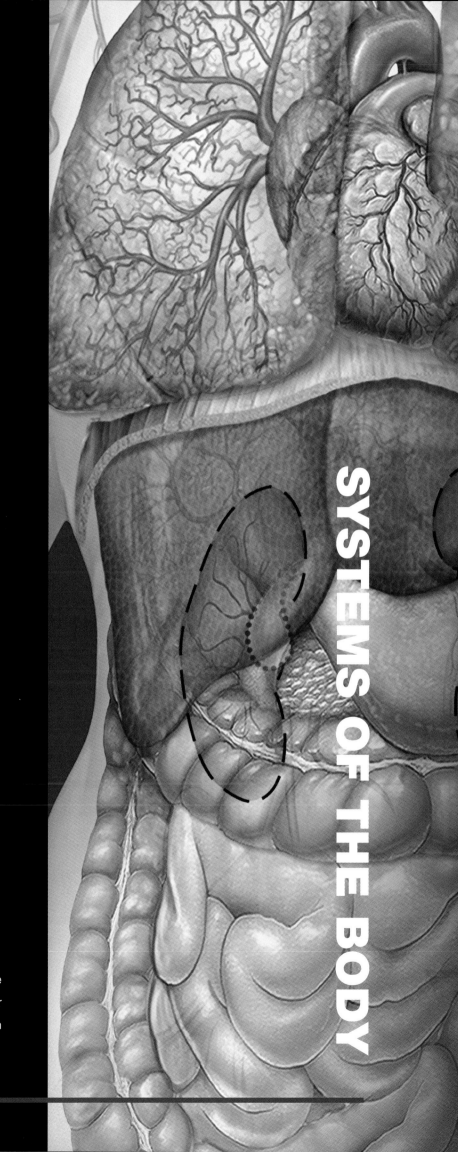

SYSTEMS OF THE BODY

• The Digestive System • The Endocrine System • The Female Reproductive System • The Lymphatic System • The Male Reproductive System • The Muscular System • The Nervous System • The Respiratory System • The Skeletal System • The Spinal Nerves • The Urinary Tract • The Vascular System and Viscera

The Digestive System

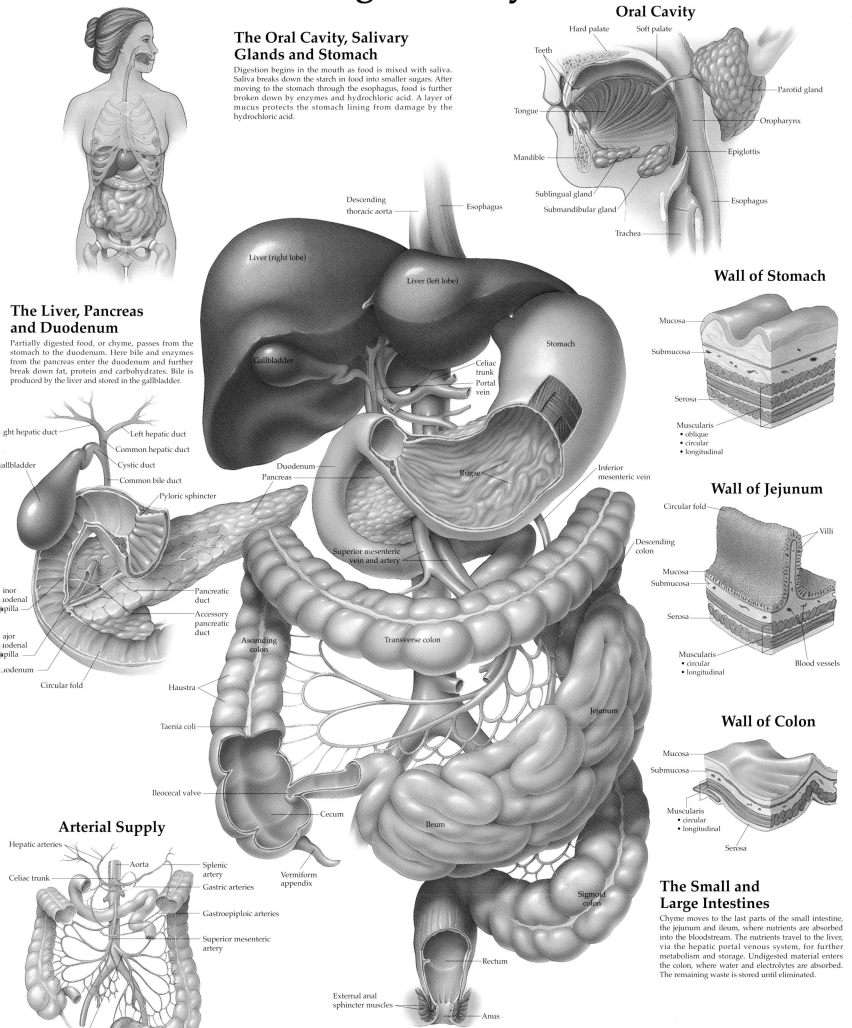

The Oral Cavity, Salivary Glands and Stomach

Digestion begins in the mouth as food is mixed with saliva. Saliva breaks down the starch in food into smaller sugars. After moving to the stomach through the esophagus, food is further broken down by enzymes and hydrochloric acid. A layer of mucus protects the stomach lining from damage by the hydrochloric acid.

Oral Cavity

Hard palate
Soft palate
Teeth
Tongue
Parotid gland
Mandible
Oropharynx
Epiglottis
Sublingual gland
Submandibular gland
Esophagus
Trachea

The Liver, Pancreas and Duodenum

Partially digested food, or chyme, passes from the stomach to the duodenum. Here bile and enzymes from the pancreas enter the duodenum and further break down fat, protein and carbohydrates. Bile is produced by the liver and stored in the gallbladder.

Descending thoracic aorta
Esophagus
Liver (right lobe)
Liver (left lobe)
Stomach
Gallbladder
Celiac trunk
Portal vein
ght hepatic duct
Left hepatic duct
Common hepatic duct
Cystic duct
allbladder
Common bile duct
Duodenum
Pancreas
Rugae
Inferior mesenteric vein
Pyloric sphincter
inor 1odenal pilla
Pancreatic duct
Accessory pancreatic duct
ajor 1odenal pilla
Superior mesenteric vein and artery
Descending colon
1odenum
Ascending colon
Transverse colon
Circular fold
Haustra
Taenia coli
Jejunum
Ileocecal valve
Cecum
Ileum
Vermiform appendix
Sigmoid colon

Wall of Stomach

Mucosa
Submucosa
Serosa
Muscularis
• oblique
• circular
• longitudinal

Wall of Jejunum

Circular fold
Villi
Mucosa
Submucosa
Serosa
Muscularis
• circular
• longitudinal
Blood vessels

Wall of Colon

Mucosa
Submucosa
Muscularis
• circular
• longitudinal
Serosa

The Small and Large Intestines

Chyme moves to the last parts of the small intestine, the jejunum and ileum, where nutrients are absorbed into the bloodstream. The nutrients travel to the liver, via the hepatic portal venous system, for further metabolism and storage. Undigested material enters the colon, where water and electrolytes are absorbed. The remaining waste is stored until eliminated.

Arterial Supply

Hepatic arteries
Aorta
Celiac trunk
Splenic artery
Gastric arteries
Gastroepiploic arteries
Superior mesenteric artery
Inferior mesenteric artery

Rectum
External anal sphincter muscles
Anus

©2014 Wolters Kluwer

The Endocrine System

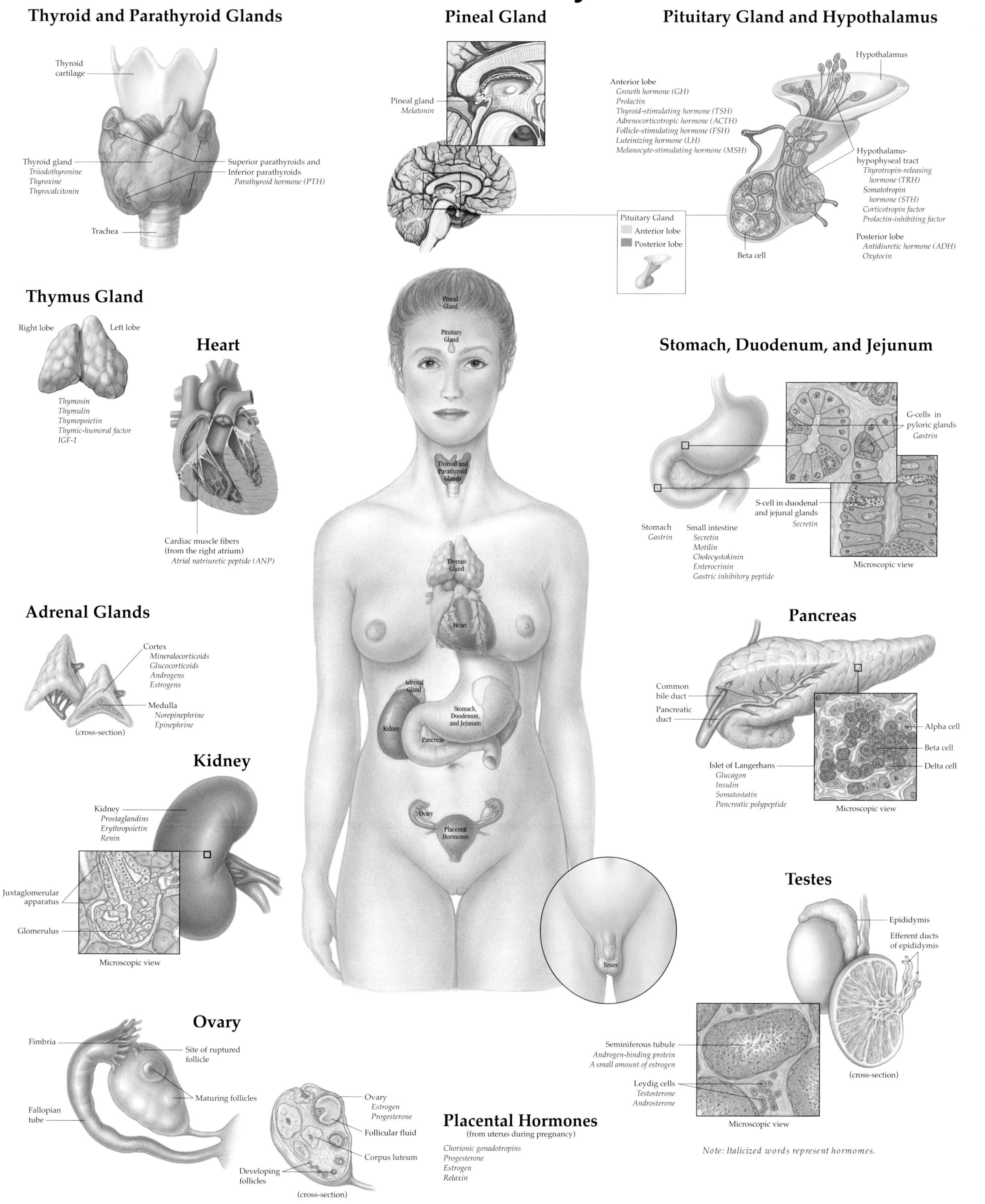

Thyroid and Parathyroid Glands

Thyroid cartilage

Thyroid gland
Triiodothyronine
Thyroxine
Thyrocalcitonin

Superior parathyroids and
Inferior parathyroids
Parathyroid hormone (PTH)

Trachea

Pineal Gland

Pineal gland
Melatonin

Pituitary Gland and Hypothalamus

Hypothalamus

Anterior lobe
Growth hormone (GH)
Prolactin
Thyroid-stimulating hormone (TSH)
Adrenocorticotropic hormone (ACTH)
Follicle-stimulating hormone (FSH)
Luteinizing hormone (LH)
Melanocyte-stimulating hormone (MSH)

Hypothalamo-hypophyseal tract
Thyrotropin-releasing hormone (TRH)
Somatotropin hormone (STH)
Corticotropin factor
Prolactin-inhibiting factor

Posterior lobe
Antidiuretic hormone (ADH)
Oxytocin

Beta cell

Pituitary Gland
Anterior lobe
Posterior lobe

Thymus Gland

Right lobe   Left lobe

Thymosin
Thymulin
Thymopoietin
Thymic-humoral factor
IGF-1

Heart

Cardiac muscle fibers
(from the right atrium)
Atrial natriuretic peptide (ANP)

Stomach, Duodenum, and Jejunum

G-cells in pyloric glands
Gastrin

S-cell in duodenal and jejunal glands
Secretin

Stomach
Gastrin

Small intestine
Secretin
Motilin
Cholecystokinin
Enterocrinin
Gastric inhibitory peptide

Microscopic view

Adrenal Glands

Cortex
Mineralocorticoids
Glucocorticoids
Androgens
Estrogens

Medulla
Norepinephrine
Epinephrine

(cross-section)

Pancreas

Common bile duct

Pancreatic duct

Islet of Langerhans
Glucagon
Insulin
Somatostatin
Pancreatic polypeptide

Alpha cell
Beta cell
Delta cell

Microscopic view

Kidney

Kidney
Prostaglandins
Erythropoietin
Renin

Juxtaglomerular apparatus

Glomerulus

Microscopic view

Testes

Epididymis

Efferent ducts of epididymis

Seminiferous tubule
Androgen-binding protein
A small amount of estrogen

Leydig cells
Testosterone
Androsterone

(cross-section)

Microscopic view

Ovary

Fimbria

Site of ruptured follicle

Maturing follicles

Fallopian tube

Ovary
Estrogen
Progesterone

Follicular fluid

Corpus luteum

Developing follicles

(cross-section)

Placental Hormones
(from uterus during pregnancy)

Chorionic gonadotropins
Progesterone
Estrogen
Relaxin

Note: Italicized words represent hormones.

Body diagram labels:
Pineal Gland
Pituitary Gland
Thyroid and Parathyroid Glands
Thymus Gland
Heart
Adrenal Gland
Stomach, Duodenum, and Jejunum
Kidney
Pancreas
Ovary
Placental Hormones
Testes

©2014 Wolters Kluwer

The Female Reproductive System

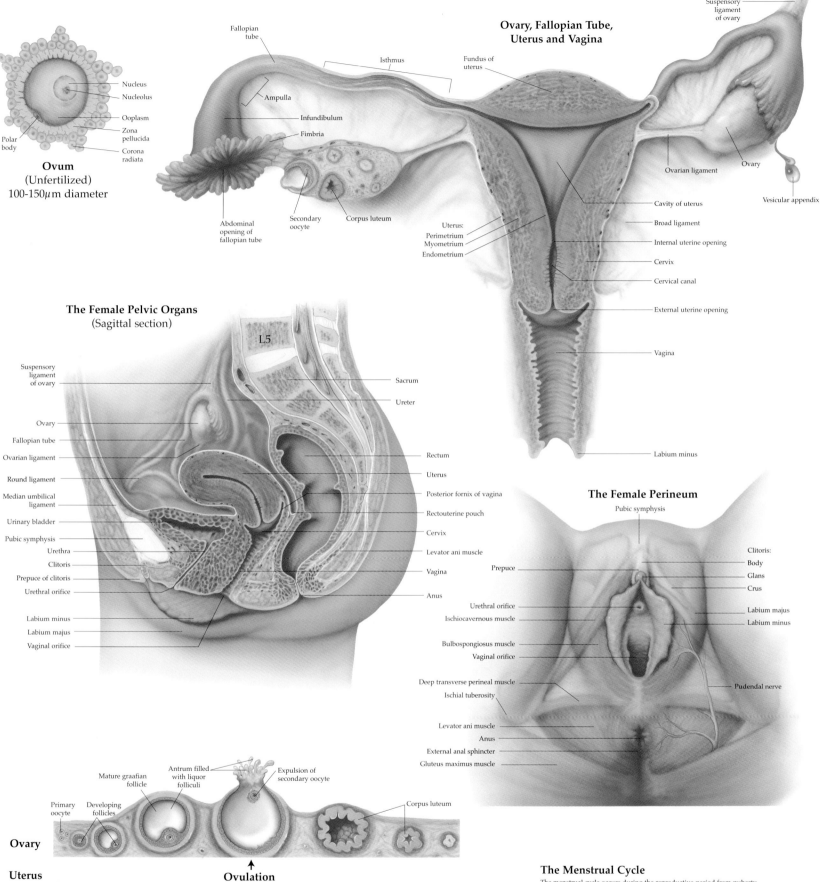

Ovum
(Unfertilized)
100-150µm diameter

- Nucleus
- Nucleolus
- Ooplasm
- Zona pellucida
- Corona radiata
- Polar body

Ovary, Fallopian Tube, Uterus and Vagina

- Fallopian tube
- Isthmus
- Ampulla
- Infundibulum
- Fimbria
- Abdominal opening of fallopian tube
- Secondary oocyte
- Corpus luteum
- Fundus of uterus
- Suspensory ligament of ovary
- Ovarian ligament
- Ovary
- Vesicular appendix
- Cavity of uterus
- Broad ligament
- Internal uterine opening
- Uterus: Perimetrium Myometrium Endometrium
- Cervix
- Cervical canal
- External uterine opening
- Vagina
- Labium minus

The Female Pelvic Organs
(Sagittal section)

- Suspensory ligament of ovary
- Ovary
- Fallopian tube
- Ovarian ligament
- Round ligament
- Median umbilical ligament
- Urinary bladder
- Pubic symphysis
- Urethra
- Clitoris
- Prepuce of clitoris
- Urethral orifice
- Labium minus
- Labium majus
- Vaginal orifice
- L5
- Sacrum
- Ureter
- Rectum
- Uterus
- Posterior fornix of vagina
- Rectouterine pouch
- Cervix
- Levator ani muscle
- Vagina
- Anus

The Female Perineum

- Pubic symphysis
- Prepuce
- Clitoris: Body Glans Crus
- Labium majus
- Labium minus
- Urethral orifice
- Ischiocavernous muscle
- Bulbospongiosus muscle
- Vaginal orifice
- Deep transverse perineal muscle
- Ischial tuberosity
- Levator ani muscle
- Anus
- External anal sphincter
- Gluteus maximus muscle
- Pudendal nerve

Ovary

- Primary oocyte
- Developing follicles
- Mature graafian follicle
- Antrum filled with liquor folliculi
- Expulsion of secondary oocyte
- Corpus luteum

Ovulation

Uterus

- Endometrium: Stratum functionale
- Uterine gland
- Stratum basale
- Myometrium
- Venous lacunae
- Endometrial vein
- Spiral artery
- Basal artery
- Arcuate artery

Day 0	4	14	26	28
Menstrual phase	Proliferative phase	Secretory phase		Premenstrual phase

The Menstrual Cycle

The menstrual cycle occurs during the reproductive period from puberty through menopause in response to rhythmic variations of hormones. The endometrial lining of the uterus proliferates in preparation for implantation of a fertilized egg. In the absence of pregnancy the lining is shed with some bleeding through the vagina.

Menopause

Menopause, the gradual interruption and cessation of menstrual cycles, occurs at about 45 to 50 years of age. It is associated with the depletion of oocytes in the ovary and subsequent decline of estrogen levels.

©2014 Wolters Kluwer

The Lymphatic System

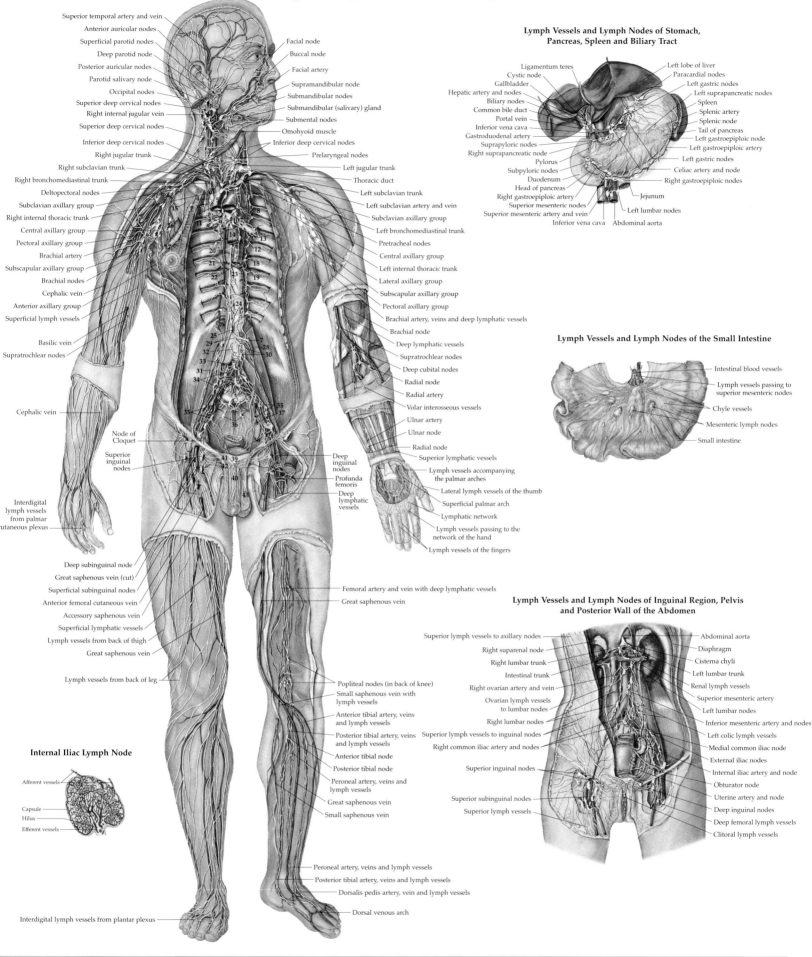

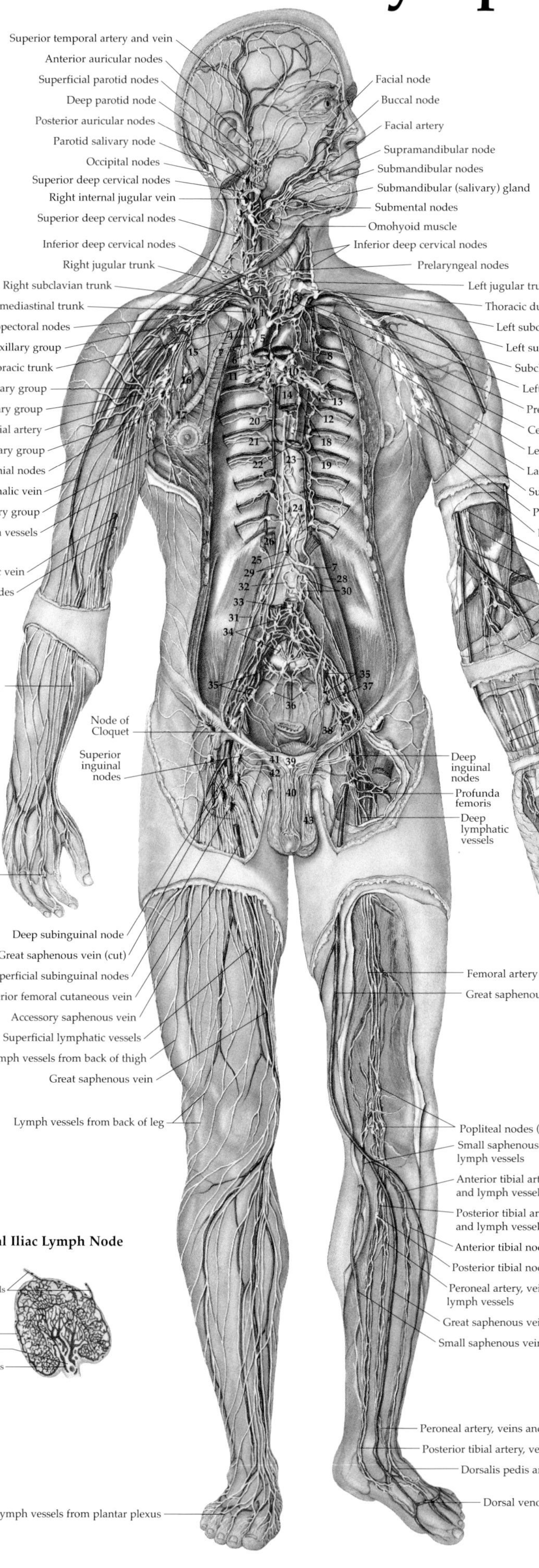
Superior temporal artery and vein
Anterior auricular nodes
Superficial parotid nodes
Deep parotid node
Posterior auricular nodes
Parotid salivary node
Occipital nodes
Superior deep cervical nodes
Right internal jugular vein
Superior deep cervical nodes
Inferior deep cervical nodes
Right jugular trunk
Right subclavian trunk
Right bronchomediastinal trunk
Deltopectoral nodes
Subclavian axillary group
Right internal thoracic trunk
Central axillary group
Pectoral axillary group
Brachial artery
Subscapular axillary group
Brachial nodes
Cephalic vein
Anterior axillary group
Superficial lymph vessels
Basilic vein
Supratrochlear nodes
Cephalic vein
Node of Cloquet
Superior inguinal nodes
Interdigital lymph vessels from palmar cutaneous plexus
Deep subinguinal node
Great saphenous vein (cut)
Superficial subinguinal nodes
Anterior femoral cutaneous vein
Accessory saphenous vein
Superficial lymphatic vessels
Lymph vessels from back of thigh
Great saphenous vein
Lymph vessels from back of leg
Interdigital lymph vessels from plantar plexus
Facial node
Buccal node
Facial artery
Supramandibular node
Submandibular nodes
Submandibular (salivary) gland
Submental nodes
Omohyoid muscle
Inferior deep cervical nodes
Prelaryngeal nodes
Left jugular trunk
Thoracic duct
Left subclavian trunk
Left subclavian artery and vein
Subclavian axillary group
Left bronchomediastinal trunk
Pretracheal nodes
Central axillary group
Left internal thoracic trunk
Lateral axillary group
Subscapular axillary group
Pectoral axillary group
Brachial artery, veins and deep lymphatic vessels
Brachial node
Deep lymphatic vessels
Supratrochlear nodes
Deep cubital nodes
Radial node
Radial artery
Volar interosseous vessels
Ulnar artery
Ulnar node
Radial node
Superior lymphatic vessels
Lymph vessels accompanying the palmar arches
Lateral lymph vessels of the thumb
Superficial palmar arch
Lymphatic network
Lymph vessels passing to the network of the hand
Lymph vessels of the fingers
Deep inguinal nodes
Profunda femoris
Deep lymphatic vessels
Femoral artery and vein with deep lymphatic vessels
Great saphenous vein
Popliteal nodes (in back of knee)
Small saphenous vein with lymph vessels
Anterior tibial artery, veins and lymph vessels
Posterior tibial artery, veins and lymph vessels
Anterior tibial node
Posterior tibial node
Peroneal artery, veins and lymph vessels
Great saphenous vein
Small saphenous vein
Peroneal artery, veins and lymph vessels
Posterior tibial artery, veins and lymph vessels
Dorsalis pedis artery, vein and lymph vessels
Dorsal venous arch

Lymph Vessels and Lymph Nodes of Stomach, Pancreas, Spleen and Biliary Tract

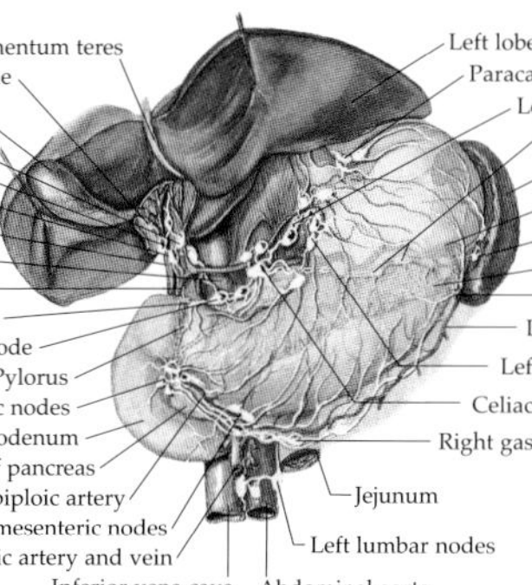
Ligamentum teres
Cystic node
Gallbladder
Hepatic artery and nodes
Biliary nodes
Common bile duct
Portal vein
Inferior vena cava
Gastroduodenal artery
Suprapyloric nodes
Right suprapancreatic node
Pylorus
Subpyloric nodes
Duodenum
Head of pancreas
Right gastroepiploic artery
Superior mesenteric nodes
Superior mesenteric artery and vein
Inferior vena cava
Abdominal aorta
Left lumbar nodes
Jejunum
Left lobe of liver
Paracardial nodes
Left gastric nodes
Left suprapancreatic nodes
Spleen
Splenic artery
Splenic node
Tail of pancreas
Left gastroepiploic node
Left gastroepiploic artery
Left gastric nodes
Celiac artery and node
Right gastroepiploic nodes

Lymph Vessels and Lymph Nodes of the Small Intestine

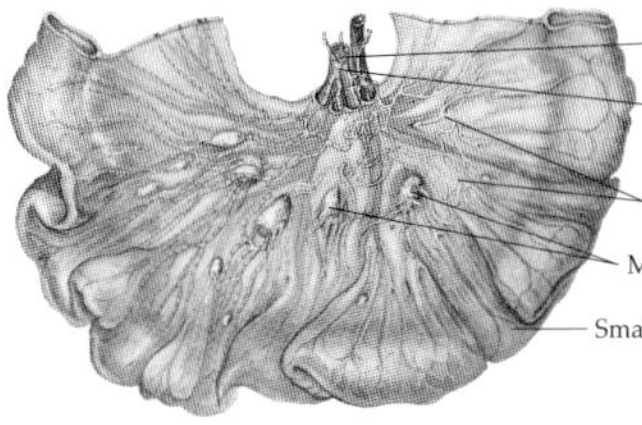
Intestinal blood vessels
Lymph vessels passing to superior mesenteric nodes
Chyle vessels
Mesenteric lymph nodes
Small intestine

Lymph Vessels and Lymph Nodes of Inguinal Region, Pelvis and Posterior Wall of the Abdomen

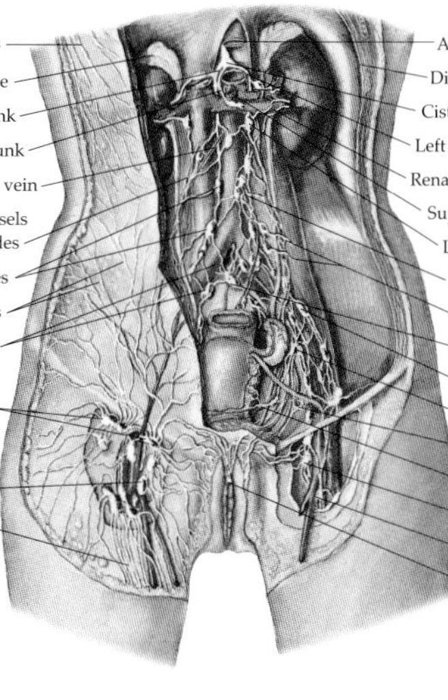
Superior lymph vessels to axillary nodes
Right suparenal node
Right lumbar trunk
Intestinal trunk
Right ovarian artery and vein
Ovarian lymph vessels to lumbar nodes
Right lumbar nodes
Superior lymph vessels to inguinal nodes
Right common iliac artery and nodes
Superior inguinal nodes
Superior subinguinal nodes
Superior lymph vessels
Abdominal aorta
Diaphragm
Cisterna chyli
Left lumbar trunk
Renal lymph vessels
Superior mesenteric artery
Left lumbar nodes
Inferior mesenteric artery and nodes
Left colic lymph vessels
Medial common iliac node
External iliac nodes
Internal iliac artery and node
Obturator node
Uterine artery and node
Deep inguinal nodes
Deep femoral lymph vessels
Clitoral lymph vessels

Internal Iliac Lymph Node

Afferent vessels
Capsule
Hilus
Efferent vessels

1. Right brachiocephalic vein
2. Left brachiocephalic vein
3. Left common carotid artery
4. Anterior superior mediastinal nodes
5. Superior vena cava
6. Right cardiac lymph branch
7. Internal thoracic node
8. Node of ligamentum arteriosum
9. Right bronchus
10. Left bronchus
11. Right tracheobronchial nodes
12. Left tracheobronchial nodes
13. Right and left bronchopulmonary nodes
14. Esophagus
15. Internal thoracic lymph vessel ending in subclavicular nodes
16. Interpectoral nodes
17. Lymph vessels from deep part of breast
18. Posterior mediastinal nodes
19. Intercostal nodes and lymph vessels
20. Azygos vein
21. Thoracic duct
22. Thoracic aorta
23. Hemiazygos vein
24. Descending right and left intercostal lymph trunks
25. Cisterna chyli
26. Right crus of diaphragm
27. Intestinal trunk
28. Psoas major muscle
29. Right and left lumbar trunks
30. Lumbar nodes
31. Testicular lymph vessels
32. Retroaortic node (lumbar nodes)
33. Preaortic node (lumbar nodes)
34. Common iliac nodes
35. Internal iliac artery and nodes
36. Sacral nodes
37. Lymph vessels to internal iliac nodes
38. Obturator vessels and nerve
39. Presymphysial node
40. Collecting lymph vessels from glans penis
41. Superior lymph vessels from the penis
42. Lymph vessels from the scrotum
43. Lymph vessels of testis and epididymus

©2014 Wolters Kluwer

The Male Reproductive System

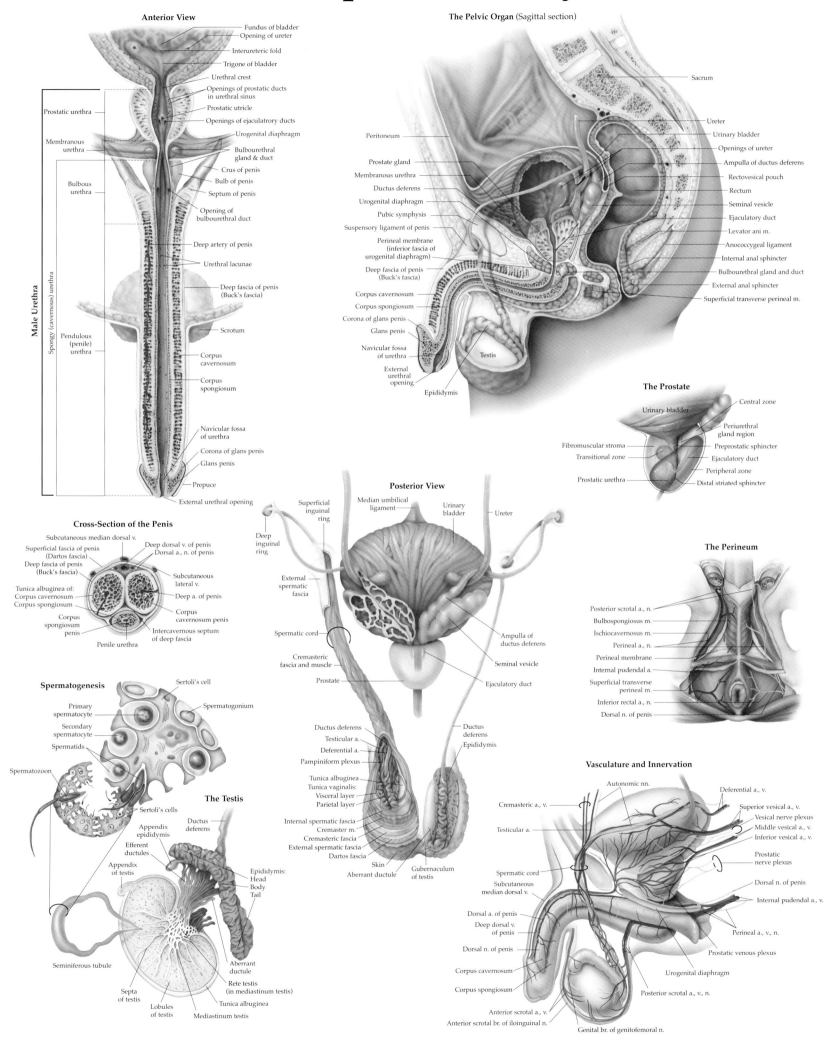

Anterior View

- Fundus of bladder
- Opening of ureter
- Int:ureteric fold
- Trigone of bladder
- Urethral crest
- Openings of prostatic ducts in urethral sinus
- Prostatic utricle
- Openings of ejaculatory ducts
- Urogenital diaphragm
- Bulbourethral gland & duct
- Crus of penis
- Bulb of penis
- Septum of penis
- Opening of bulbourethral duct
- Deep artery of penis
- Urethral lacunae
- Deep fascia of penis (Buck's fascia)
- Scrotum
- Corpus cavernosum
- Corpus spongiosum
- Navicular fossa of urethra
- Corona of glans penis
- Glans penis
- Prepuce
- External urethral opening

Prostatic urethra
Membranous urethra
Bulbous urethra
Pendulous (penile) urethra

Male Urethra
Spongy (cavernous) urethra

The Pelvic Organ (Sagittal section)

- Sacrum
- Ureter
- Urinary bladder
- Openings of ureter
- Ampulla of ductus deferens
- Rectovesical pouch
- Rectum
- Seminal vesicle
- Ejaculatory duct
- Levator ani m.
- Anococcygeal ligament
- Internal anal sphincter
- Bulbourethral gland and duct
- External anal sphincter
- Superficial transverse perineal m.
- Peritoneum
- Prostate gland
- Membranous urethra
- Ductus deferens
- Urogenital diaphragm
- Pubic symphysis
- Suspensory ligament of penis
- Perineal membrane (inferior fascia of urogenital diaphragm)
- Deep fascia of penis (Buck's fascia)
- Corpus cavernosum
- Corpus spongiosum
- Corona of glans penis
- Glans penis
- Navicular fossa of urethra
- External urethral opening
- Epididymis
- Testis

The Prostate

- Central zone
- Periurethral gland region
- Preprostatic sphincter
- Ejaculatory duct
- Peripheral zone
- Distal striated sphincter
- Urinary bladder
- Fibromuscular stroma
- Transitional zone
- Prostatic urethra

Cross-Section of the Penis

- Subcutaneous median dorsal v.
- Superficial fascia of penis (Dartos fascia)
- Deep fascia of penis (Buck's fascia)
- Tunica albuginea of: Corpus cavernosum, Corpus spongiosum
- Corpus spongiosum penis
- Penile urethra
- Deep dorsal v. of penis
- Dorsal a., n. of penis
- Subcutaneous lateral v.
- Deep a. of penis
- Corpus cavernosum penis
- Intercavernous septum of deep fascia

Posterior View

- Median umbilical ligament
- Urinary bladder
- Ureter
- Superficial inguinal ring
- Deep inguinal ring
- External spermatic fascia
- Spermatic cord
- Cremasteric fascia and muscle
- Prostate
- Ampulla of ductus deferens
- Seminal vesicle
- Ejaculatory duct

The Perineum

- Posterior scrotal a., n.
- Bulbospongiosus m.
- Ischiocavernosus m.
- Perineal a., n.
- Perineal membrane
- Internal pudendal a.
- Superficial transverse perineal m.
- Inferior rectal a., n.
- Dorsal n. of penis

Spermatogenesis

- Sertoli's cell
- Spermatogonium
- Primary spermatocyte
- Secondary spermatocyte
- Spermatids
- Spermatozoon
- Sertoli's cells

The Testis

- Ductus deferens
- Appendix epididymis
- Efferent ductules
- Appendix of testis
- Epididymis: Head, Body, Tail
- Aberrant ductule
- Rete testis (in mediastinum testis)
- Tunica albuginea
- Mediastinum testis
- Lobules of testis
- Septa of testis
- Seminiferous tubule

- Ductus deferens
- Testicular a.
- Deferential a.
- Pampiniform plexus
- Tunica albuginea
- Tunica vaginalis: Visceral layer, Parietal layer
- Internal spermatic fascia
- Cremaster m.
- Cremasteric fascia
- External spermatic fascia
- Dartos fascia
- Skin
- Aberrant ductule
- Ductus deferens
- Epididymis
- Gubernaculum of testis

Vasculature and Innervation

- Autonomic nn.
- Deferential a., v.
- Superior vesical a., v.
- Vesical nerve plexus
- Middle vesical a., v.
- Inferior vesical a., v.
- Prostatic nerve plexus
- Dorsal n. of penis
- Internal pudendal a., v.
- Perineal a., v., n.
- Prostatic venous plexus
- Urogenital diaphragm
- Posterior scrotal a., v., n.
- Genital br. of genitofemoral n.
- Cremasteric a., v.
- Testicular a.
- Spermatic cord
- Subcutaneous median dorsal v.
- Dorsal a. of penis
- Deep dorsal v. of penis
- Dorsal n. of penis
- Corpus cavernosum
- Corpus spongiosum
- Anterior scrotal a., v.
- Anterior scrotal br. of ilioinguinal n.

©2014 Wolters Kluwer

The Muscular System

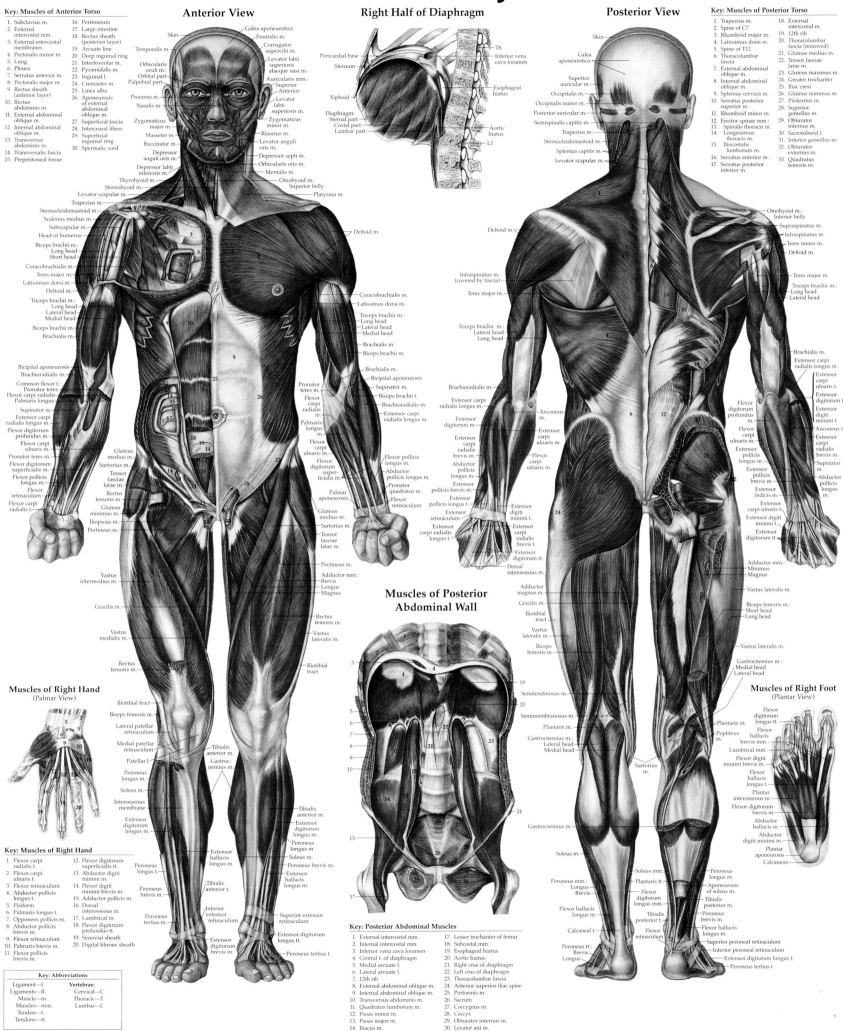

Anterior View

Right Half of Diaphragm

Posterior View

Muscles of Posterior Abdominal Wall

Muscles of Right Hand
(Palmar View)

Muscles of Right Foot
(Plantar View)

Key: Muscles of Anterior Torso

1. Subclavius m.
2. External intercostal mm.
3. External intercostal membranes
4. Pectoralis minor m.
5. Lung
6. Pleura
7. Serratus anterior m.
8. Pectoralis major m.
9. Rectus sheath (anterior layer)
10. Rectus abdominis m.
11. External abdominal oblique m.
12. Internal abdominal oblique m.
13. Transversus abdominis m.
14. Transversalis fascia
15. Preperitoneal tissue
16. Peritoneum
17. Large intestine
18. Rectus sheath (posterior layer)
19. Arcuate line
20. Deep inguinal ring
21. Interfoveolar m.
22. Pyramidalis m.
23. Inguinal l.
24. Cremaster m.
25. Linea alba
26. Aponeurosis of external abdominal oblique m.
27. Superficial fascia
28. Intercrural fibers
29. Superficial inguinal ring
30. Spermatic cord

Key: Muscles of Posterior Torso

1. Trapezius m.
2. Spine of C7
3. Rhomboid major m.
4. Latissimus dorsi m.
5. Spine of T12
6. Thoracolumbar fascia
7. External abdominal oblique m.
8. Internal abdominal oblique m.
9. Splenius cervicis m.
10. Serratus posterior superior m.
11. Rhomboid minor m.
12. Erector spinae mm.
13. Spinalis thoracis m.
14. Longissimus thoracis m.
15. Iliocostalis lumborum m.
16. Serratus anterior m.
17. Serratus posterior inferior m.
18. External intercostal m.
19. 12th rib
20. Thoracolumbar fascia (removed)
21. Gluteus medius m.
22. Tensor fasciae latae m.
23. Gluteus maximus m.
24. Greater trochanter
25. Iliac crest
26. Gluteus minimus m.
27. Piriformis m.
28. Superior gemellus m.
29. Obturator internus m.
30. Sacrotuberal l.
31. Inferior gemellus m.
32. Obturator externus m.
33. Quadratus femoris m.

Key: Muscles of Right Hand

1. Flexor carpi radialis t.
2. Flexor carpi ulnaris t.
3. Flexor retinaculum
4. Abductor pollicis longus t.
5. Pisiform
6. Palmaris longus t.
7. Opponens pollicis
8. Abductor pollicis brevis m.
9. Flexor retinaculum
10. Palmaris brevis m.
11. Flexor pollicis brevis m.
12. Flexor digitorum superficialis tt.
13. Abductor digiti minimi m.
14. Flexor digiti minimi brevis m.
15. Adductor pollicis m.
16. Dorsal interosseous m.
17. Lumbrical m.
18. Flexor digitorum profundus tt.
19. Synovial sheath
20. Digital fibrous sheath

Key: Posterior Abdominal Muscles

1. External intercostal mm.
2. Internal intercostal mm.
3. Inferior vena cava foramen
4. Central t. of diaphragm
5. Medial arcuate l.
6. Lateral arcuate l.
7. 12th rib
8. External abdominal oblique m.
9. Internal abdominal oblique m.
10. Transversus abdominis m.
11. Quadratus lumborum m.
12. Psoas minor m.
13. Psoas major m.
14. Iliacus m.
15. Inguinal l.
16. Iliopsoas m.
17. Lesser trochanter of femur
18. Subcostal mm.
19. Esophageal hiatus
20. Aortic hiatus
21. Right crus of diaphragm
22. Left crus of diaphragm
23. Thoracolumbar fascia
24. Anterior superior iliac spine
25. Piriformis m.
26. Sacrum
27. Coccygeus m.
28. Coccyx
29. Obturator internus m.
30. Levator ani m.
31. Obturator externus m.

Key: Abbreviations

Ligament—l.	Vertebrae:
Ligaments—ll.	Cervical—C
Muscle—m.	Thoracic—T
Muscles—mm.	Lumbar—L
Tendon—t.	
Tendons—tt.	

©2014 Wolters Kluwer

The Nervous System

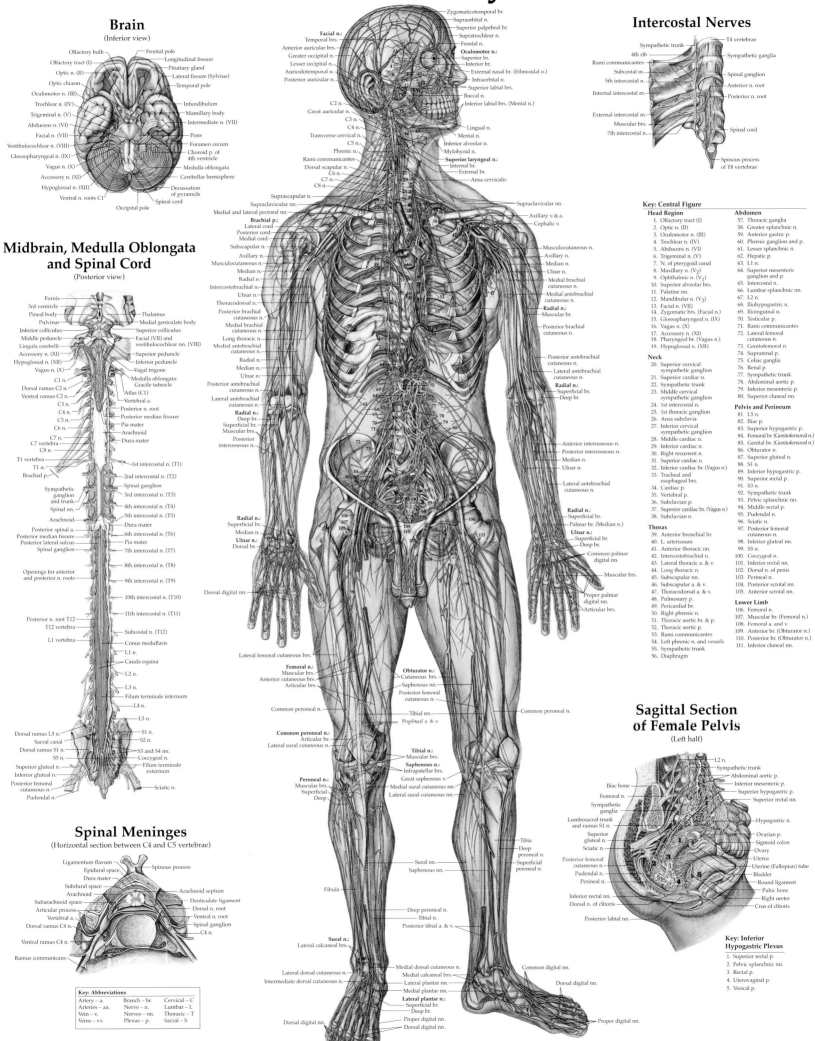

©2014 Wolters Kluwer

The Respiratory System

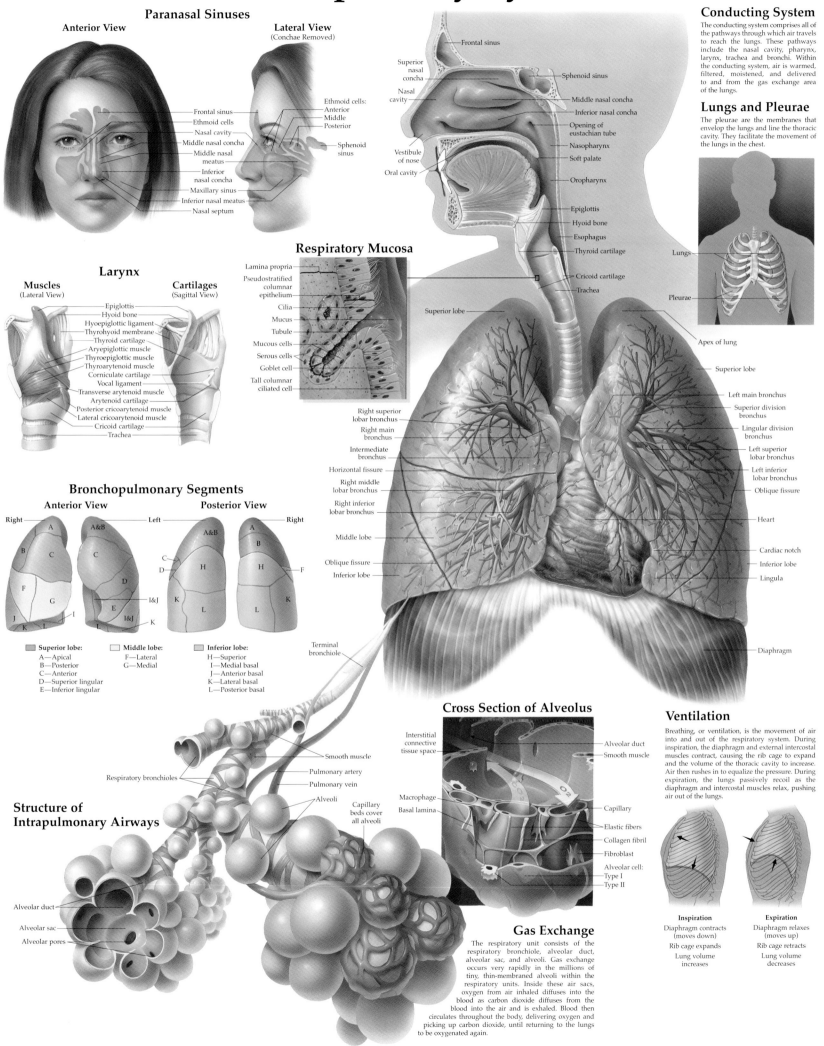

Paranasal Sinuses

Anterior View

Lateral View
(Conchae Removed)

- Frontal sinus
- Ethmoid cells
- Nasal cavity
- Middle nasal concha
- Middle nasal meatus
- Inferior nasal concha
- Maxillary sinus
- Inferior nasal meatus
- Nasal septum

Ethmoid cells:
- Anterior
- Middle
- Posterior
- Sphenoid sinus

- Frontal sinus
- Superior nasal concha
- Sphenoid sinus
- Nasal cavity
- Middle nasal concha
- Inferior nasal concha
- Opening of eustachian tube
- Nasopharynx
- Vestibule of nose
- Soft palate
- Oral cavity
- Oropharynx
- Epiglottis
- Hyoid bone
- Esophagus
- Thyroid cartilage
- Cricoid cartilage
- Trachea

Conducting System

The conducting system comprises all of the pathways through which air travels to reach the lungs. These pathways include the nasal cavity, pharynx, larynx, trachea and bronchi. Within the conducting system, air is warmed, filtered, moistened, and delivered to and from the gas exchange area of the lungs.

Lungs and Pleurae

The pleurae are the membranes that envelop the lungs and line the thoracic cavity. They facilitate the movement of the lungs in the chest.

- Lungs
- Pleurae

Larynx

Muscles
(Lateral View)

Cartilages
(Sagittal View)

- Epiglottis
- Hyoid bone
- Hyoepiglottic ligament
- Thyrohyoid membrane
- Thyroid cartilage
- Aryepiglottic muscle
- Thyroepiglottic muscle
- Thyroarytenoid muscle
- Corniculate cartilage
- Vocal ligament
- Transverse arytenoid muscle
- Arytenoid cartilage
- Posterior cricoarytenoid muscle
- Lateral cricoarytenoid muscle
- Cricoid cartilage
- Trachea

Respiratory Mucosa

- Lamina propria
- Pseudostratified columnar epithelium
- Cilia
- Mucus
- Tubule
- Mucous cells
- Serous cells
- Goblet cell
- Tall columnar ciliated cell

- Apex of lung
- Superior lobe
- Left main bronchus
- Superior division bronchus
- Lingular division bronchus
- Left superior lobar bronchus
- Left inferior lobar bronchus
- Oblique fissure
- Heart
- Cardiac notch
- Inferior lobe
- Lingula
- Diaphragm

- Superior lobe
- Right superior lobar bronchus
- Right main bronchus
- Intermediate bronchus
- Horizontal fissure
- Right middle lobar bronchus
- Right inferior lobar bronchus
- Middle lobe
- Oblique fissure
- Inferior lobe

Bronchopulmonary Segments

Anterior View

Posterior View

Right | Left | Right

Superior lobe:
- A—Apical
- B—Posterior
- C—Anterior
- D—Superior lingular
- E—Inferior lingular

Middle lobe:
- F—Lateral
- G—Medial

Inferior lobe:
- H—Superior
- I—Medial basal
- J—Anterior basal
- K—Lateral basal
- L—Posterior basal

Structure of Intrapulmonary Airways

- Terminal bronchiole
- Smooth muscle
- Respiratory bronchioles
- Pulmonary artery
- Pulmonary vein
- Alveoli
- Capillary beds cover all alveoli
- Alveolar duct
- Alveolar sac
- Alveolar pores

Cross Section of Alveolus

- Interstitial connective tissue space
- Alveolar duct
- Smooth muscle
- Macrophage
- Basal lamina
- Capillary
- Elastic fibers
- Collagen fibril
- Fibroblast
- Alveolar cell:
  - Type I
  - Type II

Ventilation

Breathing, or ventilation, is the movement of air into and out of the respiratory system. During inspiration, the diaphragm and external intercostal muscles contract, causing the rib cage to expand and the volume of the thoracic cavity to increase. Air then rushes in to equalize the pressure. During expiration, the lungs passively recoil as the diaphragm and intercostal muscles relax, pushing air out of the lungs.

Inspiration
Diaphragm contracts (moves down)
Rib cage expands
Lung volume increases

Expiration
Diaphragm relaxes (moves up)
Rib cage retracts
Lung volume decreases

Gas Exchange

The respiratory unit consists of the respiratory bronchiole, alveolar duct, alveolar sac, and alveoli. Gas exchange occurs very rapidly in the millions of tiny, thin-membraned alveoli within the respiratory units. Inside these air sacs, oxygen from air inhaled diffuses into the blood as carbon dioxide diffuses from the blood into the air and is exhaled. Blood then circulates throughout the body, delivering oxygen and picking up carbon dioxide, until returning to the lungs to be oxygenated again.

©2014 Wolters Kluwer

The Skeletal System

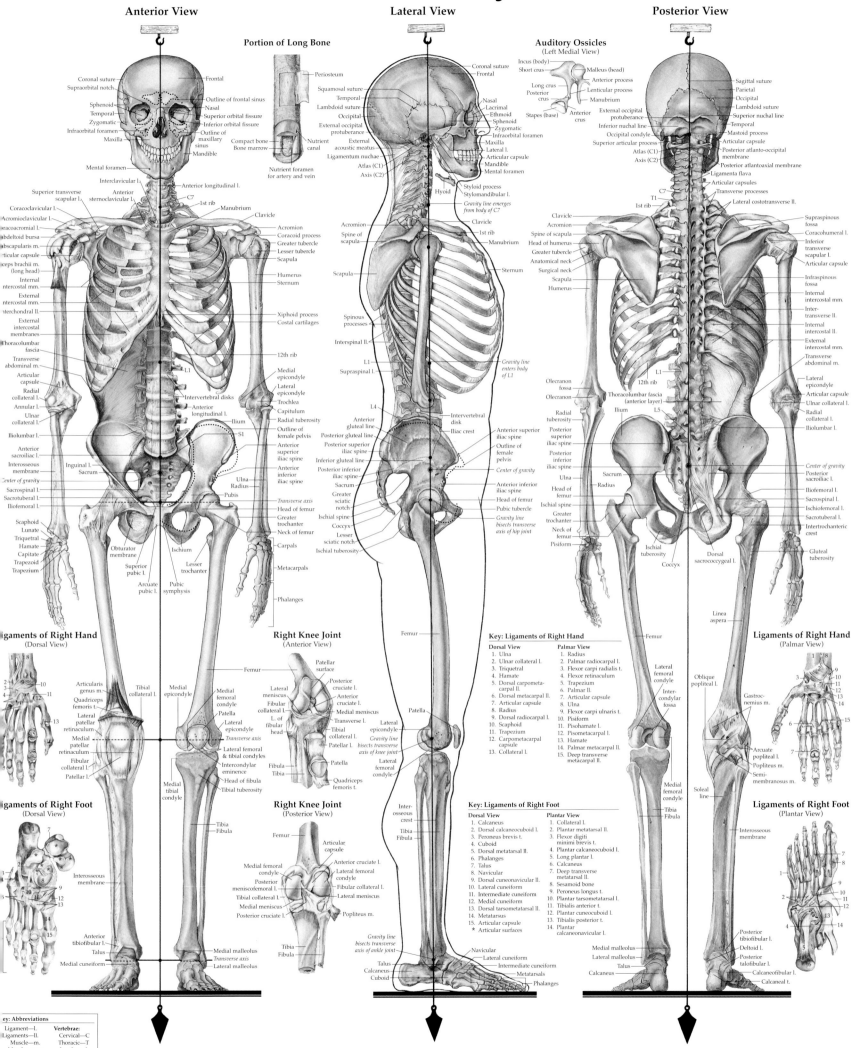

©2014 Wolters Kluwer

The Spinal Nerves

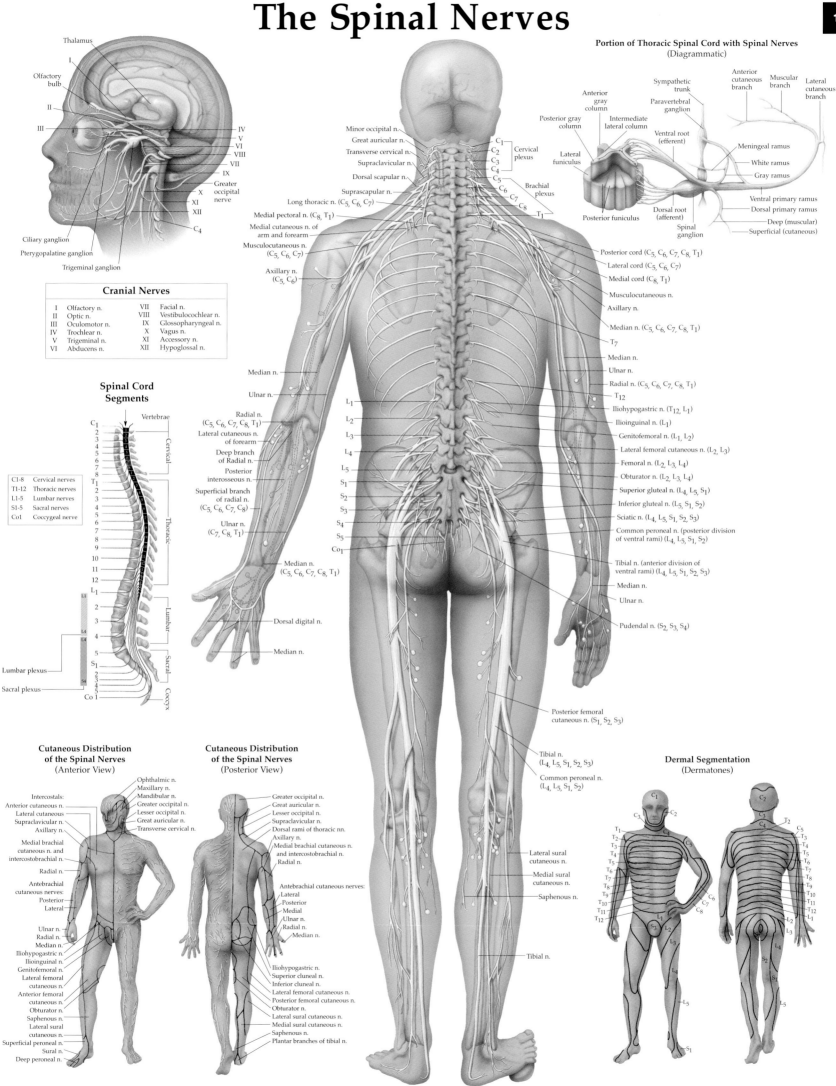

©2014 Wolters Kluwer

The Urinary Tract

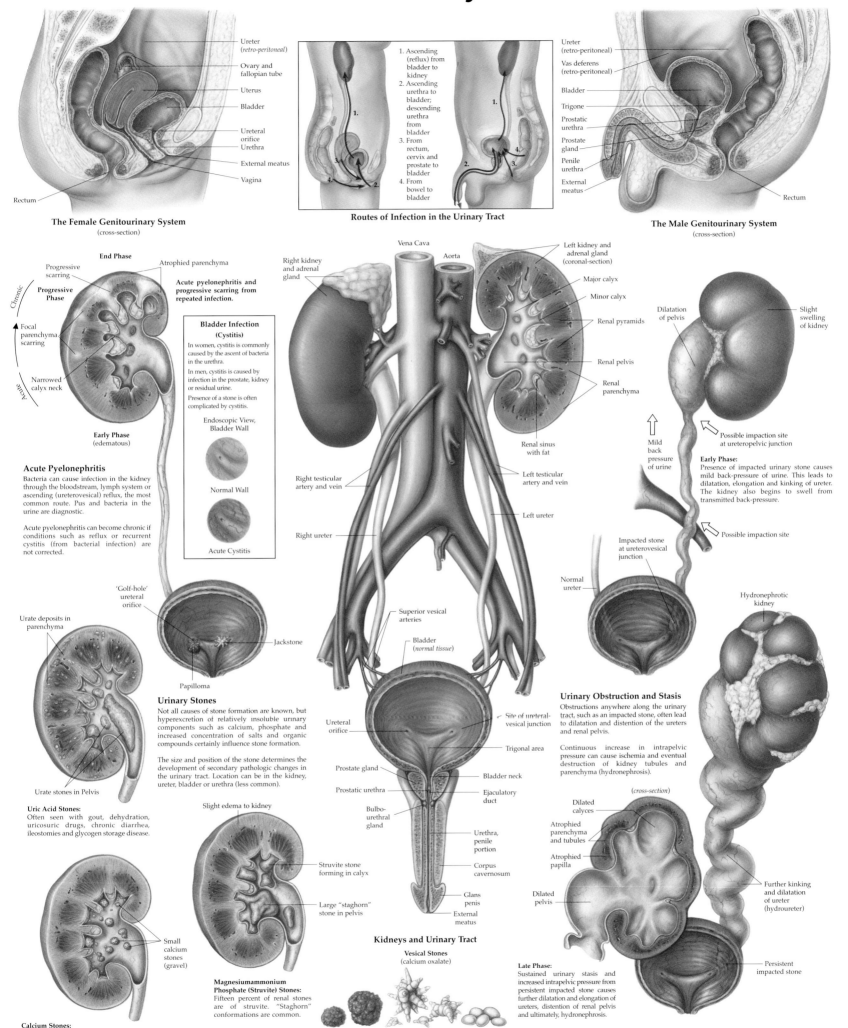

The Female Genitourinary System
(cross-section)

- Ureter (*retro-peritoneal*)
- Ovary and fallopian tube
- Uterus
- Bladder
- Ureteral orifice
- Urethra
- External meatus
- Vagina
- Rectum

Routes of Infection in the Urinary Tract

1. Ascending (reflux) from bladder to kidney
2. Ascending urethra to bladder; descending urethra from bladder
3. From rectum, cervix and prostate to bladder
4. From bowel to bladder

The Male Genitourinary System
(cross-section)

- Ureter (retro-peritoneal)
- Vas deferens (retro-peritoneal)
- Bladder
- Trigone
- Prostatic urethra
- Prostate gland
- Penile urethra
- External meatus
- Rectum

Acute Pyelonephritis

- End Phase
- Progressive scarring
- Atrophied parenchyma
- Progressive Phase
- Chronic
- Focal parenchyma scarring
- Narrowed calyx neck
- Acute
- Early Phase (edematous)

Acute pyelonephritis and progressive scarring from repeated infection.

Bacteria can cause infection in the kidney through the bloodstream, lymph system or ascending (ureterovesical) reflux, the most common route. Pus and bacteria in the urine are diagnostic.

Acute pyelonephritis can become chronic if conditions such as reflux or recurrent cystitis (from bacterial infection) are not corrected.

Bladder Infection (Cystitis)

In women, cystitis is commonly caused by the ascent of bacteria in the urethra.

In men, cystitis is caused by infection in the prostate, kidney or residual urine.

Presence of a stone is often complicated by cystitis.

Endoscopic View, Bladder Wall

- Normal Wall
- Acute Cystitis

Urinary Stones

- Urate deposits in parenchyma
- 'Golf-hole' ureteral orifice
- Jackstone
- Papilloma
- Urate stones in Pelvis

Not all causes of stone formation are known, but hyperexcretion of relatively insoluble urinary components such as calcium, phosphate and increased concentration of salts and organic compounds certainly influence stone formation.

The size and position of the stone determines the development of secondary pathologic changes in the urinary tract. Location can be in the kidney, ureter, bladder or urethra (less common).

Uric Acid Stones:
Often seen with gout, dehydration, uricosuric drugs, chronic diarrhea, ileostomies and glycogen storage disease.

- Small calcium stones (gravel)

Calcium Stones:
Seventy percent of renal stones are of calciumoxalate or mixtures of calciumoxalate and calciumphosphate in the form of hypoxyapatite. Two-thirds of patients with primary hyperparathyroidism have calcium stones.

- Slight edema to kidney
- Struvite stone forming in calyx
- Large "staghorn" stone in pelvis

Magnesiumammonium Phosphate (Struvite) Stones:
Fifteen percent of renal stones are of struvite. "Staghorn" conformations are common.

Kidneys and Urinary Tract

- Vena Cava
- Aorta
- Right kidney and adrenal gland
- Left kidney and adrenal gland (coronal-section)
- Major calyx
- Minor calyx
- Renal pyramids
- Renal pelvis
- Renal parenchyma
- Renal sinus with fat
- Right testicular artery and vein
- Left testicular artery and vein
- Left ureter
- Right ureter
- Superior vesical arteries
- Bladder (*normal tissue*)
- Ureteral orifice
- Site of ureteral-vesical junction
- Trigonal area
- Prostate gland
- Bladder neck
- Prostatic urethra
- Ejaculatory duct
- Bulbo-urethral gland
- Urethra, penile portion
- Corpus cavernosum
- Glans penis
- External meatus

Vesical Stones
(calcium oxalate)

- "Mulberries"
- "Jackstones" (*actual size*)
- "Gravel"

Urinary Obstruction and Stasis

- Dilatation of pelvis
- Slight swelling of kidney
- Mild back pressure of urine
- Possible impaction site at ureteropelvic junction

Early Phase:
Presence of impacted urinary stone causes mild back-pressure of urine. This leads to dilatation, elongation and kinking of ureter. The kidney also begins to swell from transmitted back-pressure.

- Impacted stone at ureterovesical junction
- Normal ureter
- Possible impaction site
- Hydronephrotic kidney

Obstructions anywhere along the urinary tract, such as an impacted stone, often lead to dilatation and distention of the ureters and renal pelvis.

Continuous increase in intrapelvic pressure can cause ischemia and eventual destruction of kidney tubules and parenchyma (hydronephrosis).

(*cross-section*)

- Dilated calyces
- Atrophied parenchyma and tubules
- Atrophied papilla
- Dilated pelvis
- Further kinking and dilatation of ureter (hydroureter)
- Persistent impacted stone

Late Phase:
Sustained urinary stasis and increased intrapelvic pressure from persistent impacted stone causes further dilatation and elongation of ureters, distention of renal pelvis and ultimately, hydronephrosis.

©2014 Wolters Kluwer

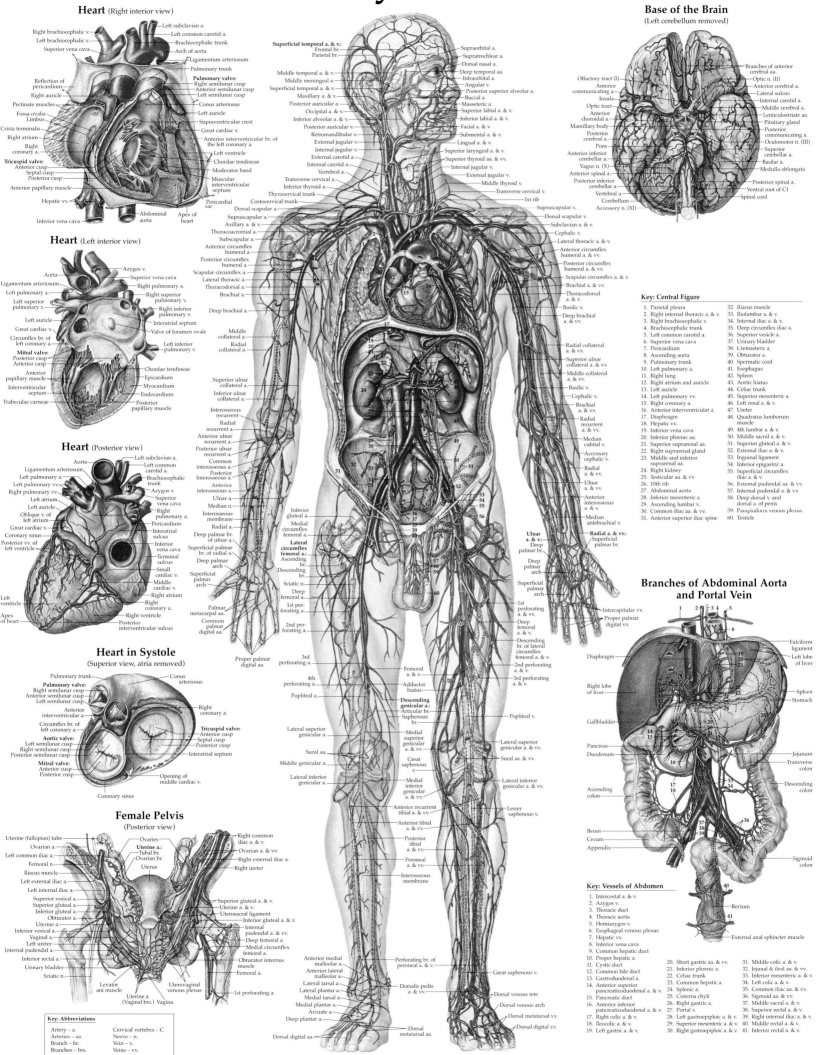

©2014 Wolters Kluwer

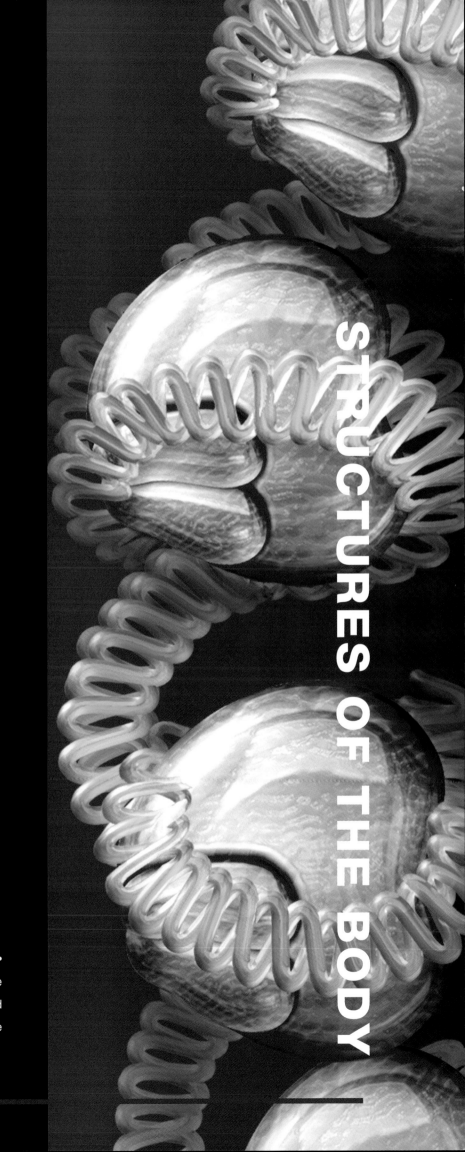

STRUCTURES OF THE BODY

The Brain

Arteries of the Brain
(Lateral View)

- Central a.
- Precentral a.
- Ascending frontal a.
- Lateral orbito-frontal a.
- Middle cerebral a.
- Anterior temporal a.
- Middle temporal a.
- Basilar a.
- Internal carotid a.
- Anterior spinal a.
- Anterior parietal a.
- Posterior parietal a.
- Angular a.
- Posterior temporal a.
- Anterior inferior cerebellar a.
- Posterior inferior cerebellar a.
- Vertebral a.

Base of Brain
(Cranial Nerves)

- Eyeball
- Olfactory bulb
- Optic n. (II)
- Olfactory tract (I)
- Optic chiasm
- Lateral olfactory stria
- Trigeminal n. (V):
- Ophthalmic n. (V₁)
- Maxillary n. (V₂)
- Mandibular n. (V₃)
- Trigeminal ganglion
- Pons
- Hypoglossal n. (XII)
- Vagus n. (X)
- Accessory n. (XI)
- Optic tract
- Oculomotor n. (III)
- Trochlear n. (IV)
- Abducens n. (VI)
- Facial n. (VII)
- Vestibulocochlear n. (VIII)
- Glossopharyngeal n. (IX)
- Medulla oblongata
- Ventral root of 1st spinal n.
- Spinal cord

Lobes of the Brain

- Cerebrum
- Cerebellum

Key
- Frontal lobe
- Parietal lobe
- Temporal lobe
- Occipital lobe

Arteries of the Brain
(Sagittal Section)

- Medial frontal branches:
- Posterior
- Middle
- Anterior
- Calloso-marginal a.
- Frontopolar a.
- Anterior cerebral a.
- Medial orbitofrontal a.
- Internal carotid a.
- Pituitary gland
- Posterior communicating a.
- Paracentral a.
- Precuneal a.
- Corpus callosum
- Posterior pericallosal a.
- Parieto-occipital a.
- Pineal body
- Calcarine a.
- Posterior cerebral a.

Limbic System

- Cingulate gyrus
- Corpus callosum
- Body of fornix
- Stria medullaris thalami
- Stria terminalis
- Mamillary body
- Olfactory tract
- Amygdala
- Hippocampus

Base of Brain
(Vessels)

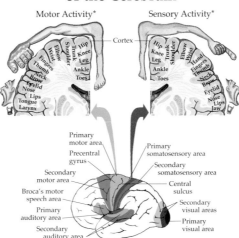

- Medial orbitofrontal a.
- Anterior communicating a.
- Middle cerebral a.
- Internal carotid a.
- Posterior communicating a.
- Posterior cerebral a.
- Anterior cerebral a.
- Superior cerebellar a.
- Pontine aa.
- Basilar a.
- Internal acoustic a.
- Anterior inferior cerebellar a.
- Vertebral a.
- Anterior spinal a.
- Posterior spinal a.
- Transverse sinus

Ventricles of the Brain
(Lateral View)

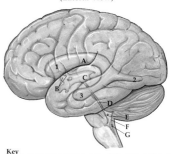

Axial view

Key
- A. Lateral ventricle:
  - 1. Anterior horn
  - 2. Posterior horn
  - 3. Inferior horn
- B. Interventricular foramen (Monro)
- C. Third ventricle
- D. Cerebral aqueduct
- E. Lateral aperture (Luschka)
- F. Fourth ventricle
- G. Median aperture (Magendie)

Coronal Section

- Longitudinal cerebral fissure
- White matter
- Corpus callosum
- Caudate nucleus
- Thalamus
- Claustrum
- Hippocampus
- Pons
- Choroid plexus of 4th ventricle
- Medulla oblongata
- Cerebral cortex (gray matter)
- Lateral ventricle
- Lateral sulcus
- Lentiform nucleus
- 3rd ventricle
- Optic tract
- Interpeduncular cistern
- Cerebellum

Circle of Willis

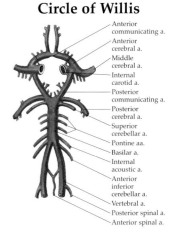

- Anterior communicating a.
- Anterior cerebral a.
- Middle cerebral a.
- Internal carotid a.
- Posterior communicating a.
- Posterior cerebral a.
- Superior cerebellar a.
- Pontine aa.
- Basilar a.
- Internal acoustic a.
- Anterior inferior cerebellar a.
- Vertebral a.
- Posterior spinal a.
- Anterior spinal a.

Circulation of Cerebrospinal Fluid (CSF)

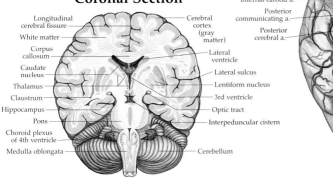

Choroid plexuses located in the lateral (A), third (B), and fourth (C) ventricles constantly produce CSF. The fluid circulates through the ventricles and foramina of the brain and within the subarachnoid space surrounding the brain and spinal cord. CSF drains into the venous blood by passing through arachnoid granulations located in the dura mater just above the brain (D). Arrows in the adjacent illustration demonstrate the flow of CSF.

Key: Abbreviations
- Artery—a.
- Arteries—aa.
- Nerve—n.

Somatotopic Organization of the Cerebrum

Motor Activity*
Sensory Activity*

- Cortex
- Hip, Knee, Trunk, Shoulder, Elbow, Wrist, Hand, Fingers, Thumb, Leg, Ankle, Toes, Neck, Brow, Eyelid, Nose, Lips, Tongue, Larynx
- Primary motor area
- Precentral gyrus
- Secondary motor area
- Broca's motor speech area
- Primary auditory area
- Secondary auditory area
- Primary somatosensory area
- Secondary somatosensory area
- Central sulcus
- Secondary visual areas
- Primary visual area

* The exaggerated caricatures sprawling over the illustrations above represent approximate centers within the brain for sensory and motor activities of the named body parts.

Meninges of the Brain

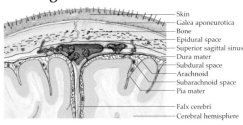

- Skin
- Galea aponeurotica
- Bone
- Epidural space
- Superior sagittal sinus
- Dura mater
- Subdural space
- Arachnoid
- Subarachnoid space
- Pia mater
- Falx cerebri
- Cerebral hemisphere

©2014 Wolters Kluwer

The Ear - Organs of Hearing and Balance

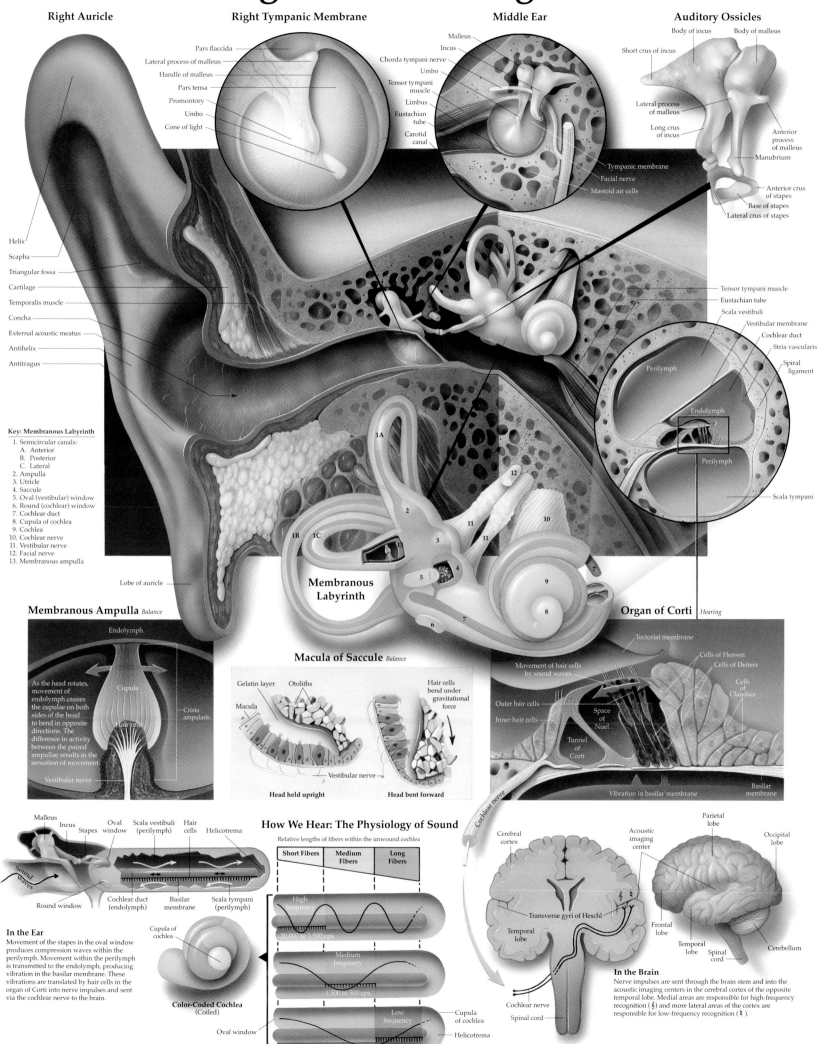

Right Auricle

- Helix
- Scapha
- Triangular fossa
- Cartilage
- Temporalis muscle
- Concha
- External acoustic meatus
- Antihelix
- Antitragus

Key: Membranous Labyrinth

1. Semicircular canals:
   A. Anterior
   B. Posterior
   C. Lateral
2. Ampulla
3. Utricle
4. Saccule
5. Oval (vestibular) window
6. Round (cochlear) window
7. Cochlear duct
8. Cupula of cochlea
9. Cochlea
10. Cochlear nerve
11. Vestibular nerve
12. Facial nerve
13. Membranous ampulla

- Lobe of auricle

Right Tympanic Membrane

- Pars flaccida
- Lateral process of malleus
- Handle of malleus
- Pars tensa
- Promontory
- Umbo
- Cone of light

Middle Ear

- Malleus
- Incus
- Chorda tympani nerve
- Umbo
- Tensor tympani muscle
- Limbus
- Eustachian tube
- Carotid canal
- Tympanic membrane
- Facial nerve
- Mastoid air cells

Auditory Ossicles

- Body of incus
- Body of malleus
- Short crus of incus
- Lateral process of malleus
- Long crus of incus
- Anterior process of malleus
- Manubrium
- Anterior crus of stapes
- Base of stapes
- Lateral crus of stapes

- Tensor tympani muscle
- Eustachian tube
- Scala vestibuli
- Vestibular membrane
- Cochlear duct
- Stria vascularis
- Spiral ligament
- Perilymph
- Endolymph
- Perilymph
- Scala tympani

Membranous Labyrinth

Membranous Ampulla *Balance*

Endolymph

As the head rotates, movement of endolymph causes the cupulae on both sides of the head to bend in opposite directions. The difference in activity between the paired ampullae results in the sensation of movement.

- Cupula
- Crista ampularis
- Hair cells
- Vestibular nerve

Macula of Saccule *Balance*

- Gelatin layer
- Otoliths
- Macula
- Hair cells bend under gravitational force
- Vestibular nerve

Head held upright   **Head bent forward**

Organ of Corti *Hearing*

- Tectorial membrane
- Movement of hair cells by sound waves
- Cells of Hensen
- Cells of Deiters
- Cells of Claudius
- Outer hair cells
- Inner hair cells
- Space of Nuel
- Tunnel of Corti
- Vibration in basilar membrane
- Basilar membrane

In the Ear

Movement of the stapes in the oval window produces compression waves within the perilymph. Movement within the perilymph is transmitted to the endolymph, producing vibration in the basilar membrane. These vibrations are translated by hair cells in the organ of Corti into nerve impulses and sent via the cochlear nerve to the brain.

- Malleus
- Incus
- Stapes
- Oval window
- Scala vestibuli (perilymph)
- Hair cells
- Helicotrema
- Sound Waves
- Round window
- Cochlear duct (endolymph)
- Basilar membrane
- Scala tympani (perilymph)

- Cupula of cochlea
- **Color-Coded Cochlea** (Coiled)
- Oval window
- Round window

How We Hear: The Physiology of Sound

Relative lengths of fibers within the unwound cochlea

Short Fibers	Medium Fibers	Long Fibers

- High frequency — 20,000 to 1,500 cps
- Medium frequency — 1,500 to 500 cps
- Low frequency — 500 to 20 cps
- Cupula of cochlea
- Helicotrema

In the Brain

Nerve impulses are sent through the brain stem and into the acoustic imaging centers in the cerebral cortex of the opposite temporal lobe. Medial areas are responsible for high-frequency recognition (𝄞) and more lateral areas of the cortex are responsible for low-frequency recognition (𝄢).

- Cerebral cortex
- Acoustic imaging center
- Parietal lobe
- Occipital lobe
- Transverse gyri of Heschl
- Temporal lobe
- Frontal lobe
- Temporal lobe
- Spinal cord
- Cerebellum
- Cochlear nerve
- Cochlear nerve
- Spinal cord

©2014 Wolters Kluwer

Ear, Nose and Throat

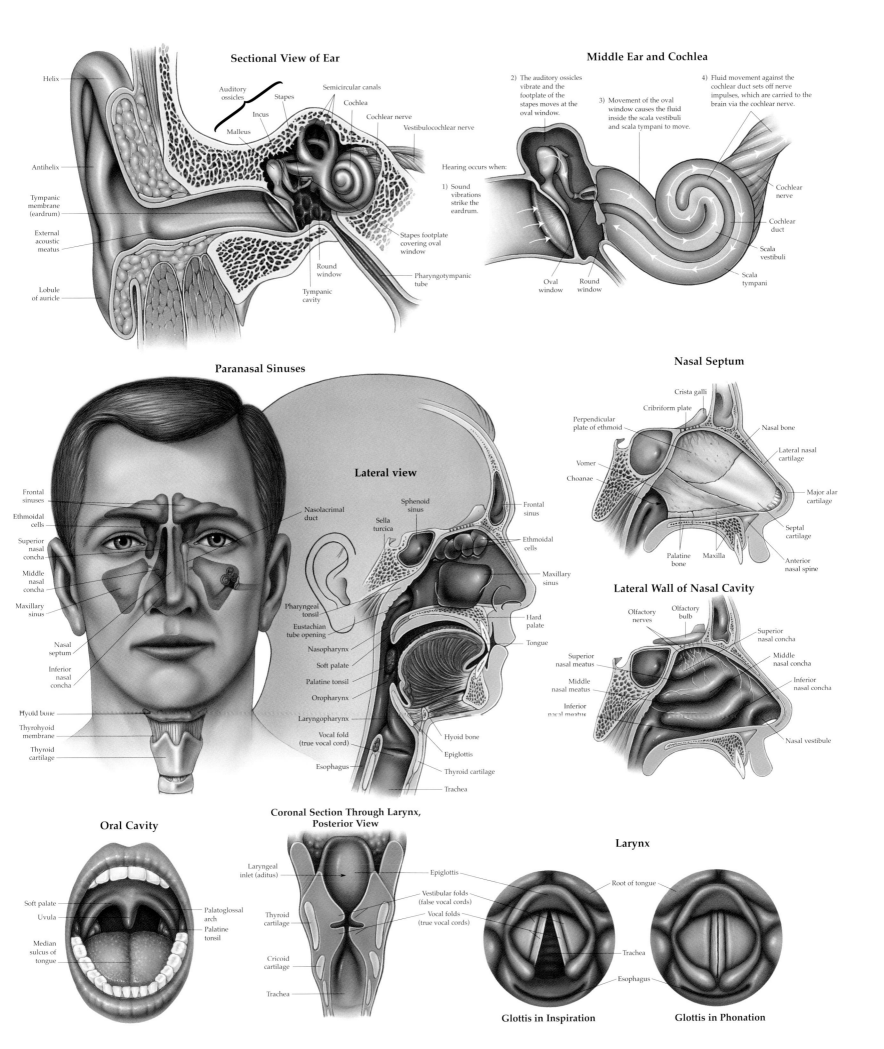

Sectional View of Ear

Helix
Antihelix
Tympanic membrane (eardrum)
External acoustic meatus
Lobule of auricle
Auditory ossicles
Stapes
Incus
Malleus
Semicircular canals
Cochlea
Cochlear nerve
Vestibulocochlear nerve
Stapes footplate covering oval window
Round window
Tympanic cavity
Pharyngotympanic tube

Middle Ear and Cochlea

2) The auditory ossicles vibrate and the footplate of the stapes moves at the oval window.

3) Movement of the oval window causes the fluid inside the scala vestibuli and scala tympani to move.

4) Fluid movement against the cochlear duct sets off nerve impulses, which are carried to the brain via the cochlear nerve.

Hearing occurs when:

1) Sound vibrations strike the eardrum.

Cochlear nerve
Cochlear duct
Scala vestibuli
Scala tympani
Oval window
Round window

Paranasal Sinuses

Frontal sinuses
Ethmoidal cells
Superior nasal concha
Middle nasal concha
Maxillary sinus
Nasal septum
Inferior nasal concha
Hyoid bone
Thyrohyoid membrane
Thyroid cartilage

Lateral view

Nasolacrimal duct
Sella turcica
Sphenoid sinus
Frontal sinus
Ethmoidal cells
Maxillary sinus
Hard palate
Tongue
Pharyngeal tonsil
Eustachian tube opening
Nasopharynx
Soft palate
Palatine tonsil
Oropharynx
Laryngopharynx
Vocal fold (true vocal cord)
Esophagus
Hyoid bone
Epiglottis
Thyroid cartilage
Trachea

Nasal Septum

Crista galli
Cribriform plate
Perpendicular plate of ethmoid
Vomer
Choanae
Nasal bone
Lateral nasal cartilage
Major alar cartilage
Septal cartilage
Palatine bone
Maxilla
Anterior nasal spine

Lateral Wall of Nasal Cavity

Olfactory nerves
Olfactory bulb
Superior nasal meatus
Middle nasal meatus
Inferior nasal meatus
Superior nasal concha
Middle nasal concha
Inferior nasal concha
Nasal vestibule

Oral Cavity

Soft palate
Uvula
Median sulcus of tongue
Palatoglossal arch
Palatine tonsil

Coronal Section Through Larynx, Posterior View

Laryngeal inlet (aditus)
Thyroid cartilage
Cricoid cartilage
Trachea
Epiglottis
Vestibular folds (false vocal cords)
Vocal folds (true vocal cords)

Larynx

Root of tongue
Trachea
Esophagus

Glottis in Inspiration

Glottis in Phonation

©2014 Wolters Kluwer

The Eye

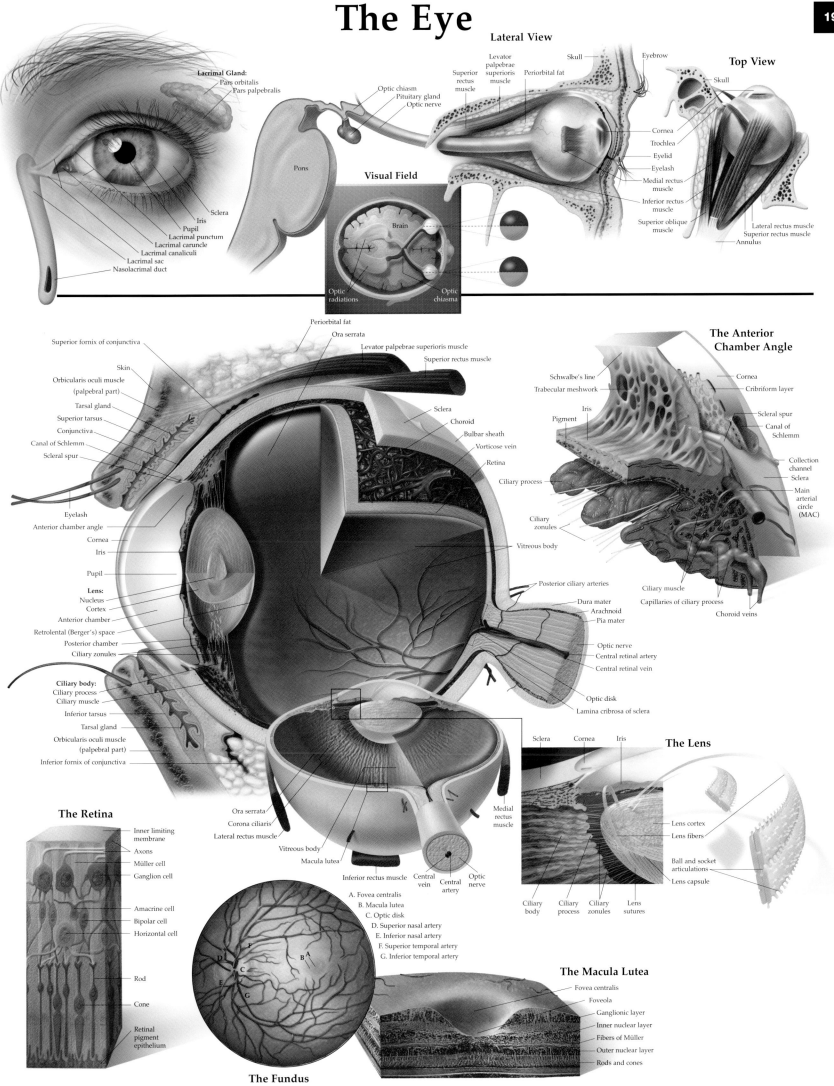

Lacrimal Gland:
Pars orbitalis
Pars palpebralis

Sclera
Iris
Pupil
Lacrimal punctum
Lacrimal caruncle
Lacrimal canaliculi
Lacrimal sac
Nasolacrimal duct

Optic chiasm
Pituitary gland
Optic nerve

Pons

Visual Field

Brain

Optic radiations
Optic chiasma

Lateral View

Levator palpebrae superioris muscle
Superior rectus muscle
Skull
Eyebrow
Periorbital fat

Cornea
Trochlea
Eyelid
Eyelash
Medial rectus muscle
Inferior rectus muscle
Superior oblique muscle

Top View

Skull

Lateral rectus muscle
Superior rectus muscle
Annulus

Superior fornix of conjunctiva
Skin
Orbicularis oculi muscle (palpebral part)
Tarsal gland
Superior tarsus
Conjunctiva
Canal of Schlemm
Scleral spur
Eyelash
Anterior chamber angle
Cornea
Iris
Pupil
Lens:
Nucleus
Cortex
Anterior chamber
Retrolental (Berger's) space
Posterior chamber
Ciliary zonules
Ciliary body:
Ciliary process
Ciliary muscle
Inferior tarsus
Tarsal gland
Orbicularis oculi muscle (palpebral part)
Inferior fornix of conjunctiva

Periorbital fat
Ora serrata
Levator palpebrae superioris muscle
Superior rectus muscle

Sclera
Choroid
Bulbar sheath
Vorticose vein
Retina

Vitreous body

Posterior ciliary arteries
Dura mater
Arachnoid
Pia mater

Optic nerve
Central retinal artery
Central retinal vein

Optic disk
Lamina cribrosa of sclera

The Anterior Chamber Angle

Schwalbe's line
Trabecular meshwork
Pigment
Iris

Cornea
Cribriform layer
Scleral spur
Canal of Schlemm
Collection channel
Sclera
Main arterial circle (MAC)

Ciliary process
Ciliary zonules
Ciliary muscle
Capillaries of ciliary process
Choroid veins

Ora serrata
Corona ciliaris
Lateral rectus muscle
Vitreous body
Macula lutea

Medial rectus muscle

Inferior rectus muscle
Central vein
Central artery
Optic nerve

A. Fovea centralis
B. Macula lutea
C. Optic disk
D. Superior nasal artery
E. Inferior nasal artery
F. Superior temporal artery
G. Inferior temporal artery

The Lens

Sclera
Cornea
Iris

Lens cortex
Lens fibers
Ball and socket articulations
Lens capsule

Ciliary body
Ciliary process
Ciliary zonules
Lens sutures

The Retina

Inner limiting membrane
Axons
Müller cell
Ganglion cell
Amacrine cell
Bipolar cell
Horizontal cell
Rod
Cone
Retinal pigment epithelium

The Fundus

The Macula Lutea

Fovea centralis
Foveola
Ganglionic layer
Inner nuclear layer
Fibers of Müller
Outer nuclear layer
Rods and cones

©2014 Wolters Kluwer

Foot and Ankle

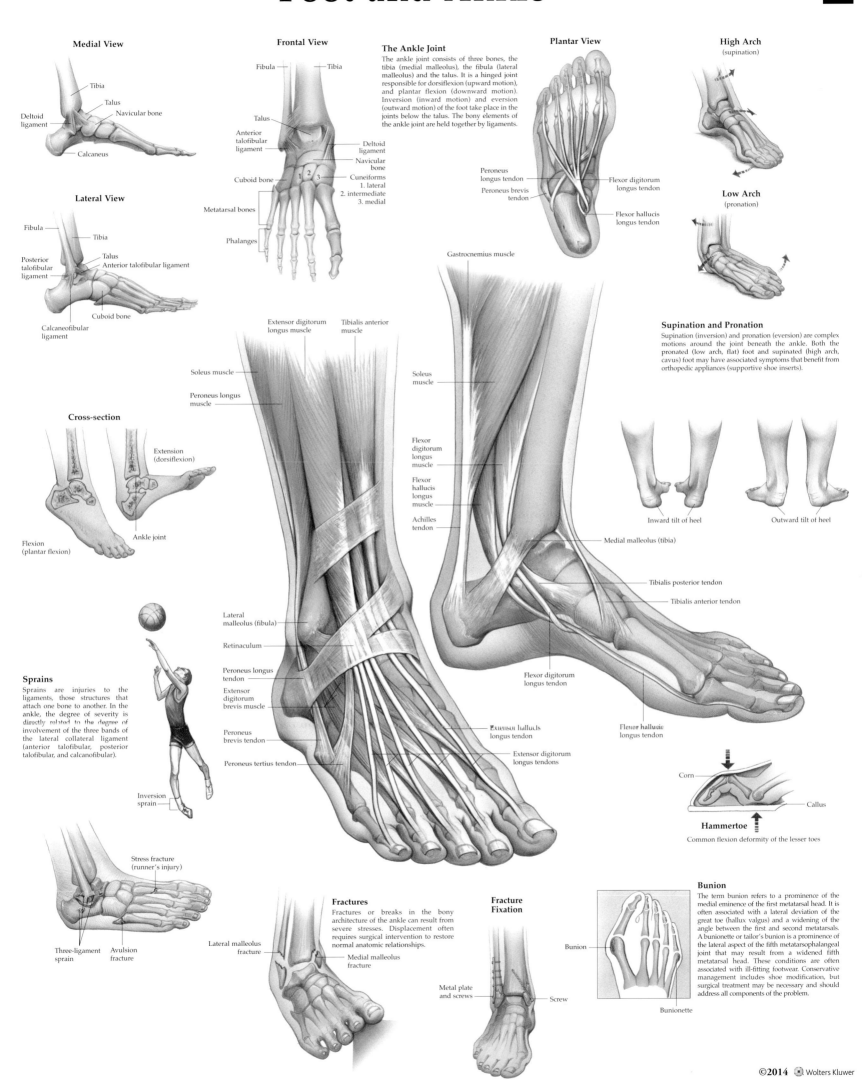

Medial View

Tibia
Talus
Navicular bone
Deltoid ligament
Calcaneus

Lateral View

Fibula
Tibia
Posterior talofibular ligament
Talus
Anterior talofibular ligament
Cuboid bone
Calcaneofibular ligament

Cross-section

Extension (dorsiflexion)
Ankle joint
Flexion (plantar flexion)

Sprains

Sprains are injuries to the ligaments, those structures that attach one bone to another. In the ankle, the degree of severity is directly related to the degree of involvement of the three bands of the lateral collateral ligament (anterior talofibular, posterior talofibular, and calcanofibular).

Inversion sprain

Stress fracture (runner's injury)

Three-ligament sprain
Avulsion fracture

Frontal View

Fibula
Tibia
Talus
Anterior talofibular ligament
Cuboid bone
Deltoid ligament
Navicular bone
1 2 3
Cuneiforms
1. lateral
2. intermediate
3. medial
Metatarsal bones
Phalanges

The Ankle Joint

The ankle joint consists of three bones, the tibia (medial malleolus), the fibula (lateral malleolus) and the talus. It is a hinged joint responsible for dorsiflexion (upward motion), and plantar flexion (downward motion). Inversion (inward motion) and eversion (outward motion) of the foot take place in the joints below the talus. The bony elements of the ankle joint are held together by ligaments.

Extensor digitorum longus muscle
Tibialis anterior muscle
Soleus muscle
Peroneus longus muscle
Lateral malleolus (fibula)
Retinaculum
Peroneus longus tendon
Extensor digitorum brevis muscle
Peroneus brevis tendon
Peroneus tertius tendon

Gastrocnemius muscle
Soleus muscle
Flexor digitorum longus muscle
Flexor hallucis longus muscle
Achilles tendon

Medial malleolus (tibia)
Tibialis posterior tendon
Tibialis anterior tendon
Flexor digitorum longus tendon
Flexor hallucis longus tendon
Extensor hallucis longus tendon
Extensor digitorum longus tendons

Plantar View

Peroneus longus tendon
Peroneus brevis tendon
Flexor digitorum longus tendon
Flexor hallucis longus tendon

High Arch (supination)

Low Arch (pronation)

Supination and Pronation

Supination (inversion) and pronation (eversion) are complex motions around the joint beneath the ankle. Both the pronated (low arch, flat) foot and supinated (high arch, cavus) foot may have associated symptoms that benefit from orthopedic appliances (supportive shoe inserts).

Inward tilt of heel
Outward tilt of heel

Corn
Callus

Hammertoe
Common flexion deformity of the lesser toes

Fractures

Fractures or breaks in the bony architecture of the ankle can result from severe stresses. Displacement often requires surgical intervention to restore normal anatomic relationships.

Lateral malleolus fracture
Medial malleolus fracture

Fracture Fixation

Metal plate and screws
Screw

Bunion

The term bunion refers to a prominence of the medial eminence of the first metatarsal head. It is often associated with a lateral deviation of the great toe (hallux valgus) and a widening of the angle between the first and second metatarsals. A bunionette or tailor's bunion is a prominence of the lateral aspect of the fifth metatarsophalangeal joint that may result from a widened fifth metatarsal head. These conditions are often associated with ill-fitting footwear. Conservative management includes shoe modification, but surgical treatment may be necessary and should address all components of the problem.

Bunion
Bunionette

©2014 Wolters Kluwer

Hand and Wrist

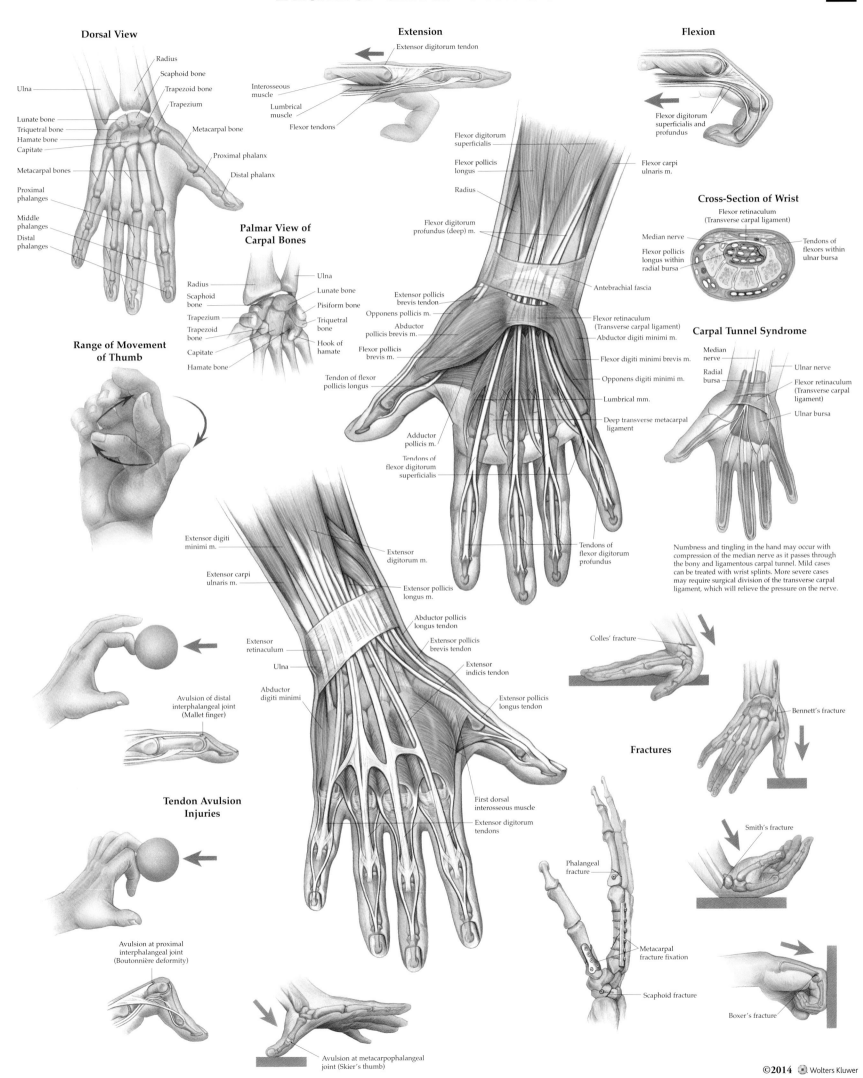

Dorsal View

Ulna
Radius
Scaphoid bone
Trapezoid bone
Trapezium
Lunate bone
Triquetral bone
Hamate bone
Capitate
Metacarpal bone
Metacarpal bones
Proximal phalanx
Distal phalanx
Proximal phalanges
Middle phalanges
Distal phalanges

Extension

Extensor digitorum tendon
Interosseous muscle
Lumbrical muscle
Flexor tendons

Flexion

Flexor digitorum superficialis and profundus

Palmar View of Carpal Bones

Radius
Scaphoid bone
Trapezium
Trapezoid bone
Capitate
Hamate bone
Ulna
Lunate bone
Pisiform bone
Triquetral bone
Hook of hamate

Range of Movement of Thumb

Flexor digitorum superficialis
Flexor pollicis longus
Radius
Flexor digitorum profundus (deep) m.
Extensor pollicis brevis tendon
Opponens pollicis m.
Abductor pollicis brevis m.
Flexor pollicis brevis m.
Tendon of flexor pollicis longus
Adductor pollicis m.
Tendons of flexor digitorum superficialis

Flexor carpi ulnaris m.

Cross-Section of Wrist

Flexor retinaculum (Transverse carpal ligament)
Median nerve
Flexor pollicis longus within radial bursa
Tendons of flexors within ulnar bursa
Antebrachial fascia

Carpal Tunnel Syndrome

Flexor retinaculum (Transverse carpal ligament)
Abductor digiti minimi m.
Flexor digiti minimi brevis m.
Opponens digiti minimi m.
Lumbrical mm.
Deep transverse metacarpal ligament
Tendons of flexor digitorum profundus

Median nerve
Radial bursa
Ulnar nerve
Flexor retinaculum (Transverse carpal ligament)
Ulnar bursa

Numbness and tingling in the hand may occur with compression of the median nerve as it passes through the bony and ligamentous carpal tunnel. Mild cases can be treated with wrist splints. More severe cases may require surgical division of the transverse carpal ligament, which will relieve the pressure on the nerve.

Extensor digiti minimi m.
Extensor carpi ulnaris m.
Extensor retinaculum
Ulna
Abductor digiti minimi
Extensor digitorum m.
Extensor pollicis longus m.
Abductor pollicis longus tendon
Extensor pollicis brevis tendon
Extensor indicis tendon
Extensor pollicis longus tendon
First dorsal interosseous muscle
Extensor digitorum tendons

Tendon Avulsion Injuries

Avulsion of distal interphalangeal joint (Mallet finger)

Avulsion at proximal interphalangeal joint (Boutonnière deformity)

Avulsion at metacarpophalangeal joint (Skier's thumb)

Fractures

Colles' fracture
Bennett's fracture
Smith's fracture
Phalangeal fracture
Metacarpal fracture fixation
Scaphoid fracture
Boxer's fracture

©2014 Wolters Kluwer

Anatomy of the Heart

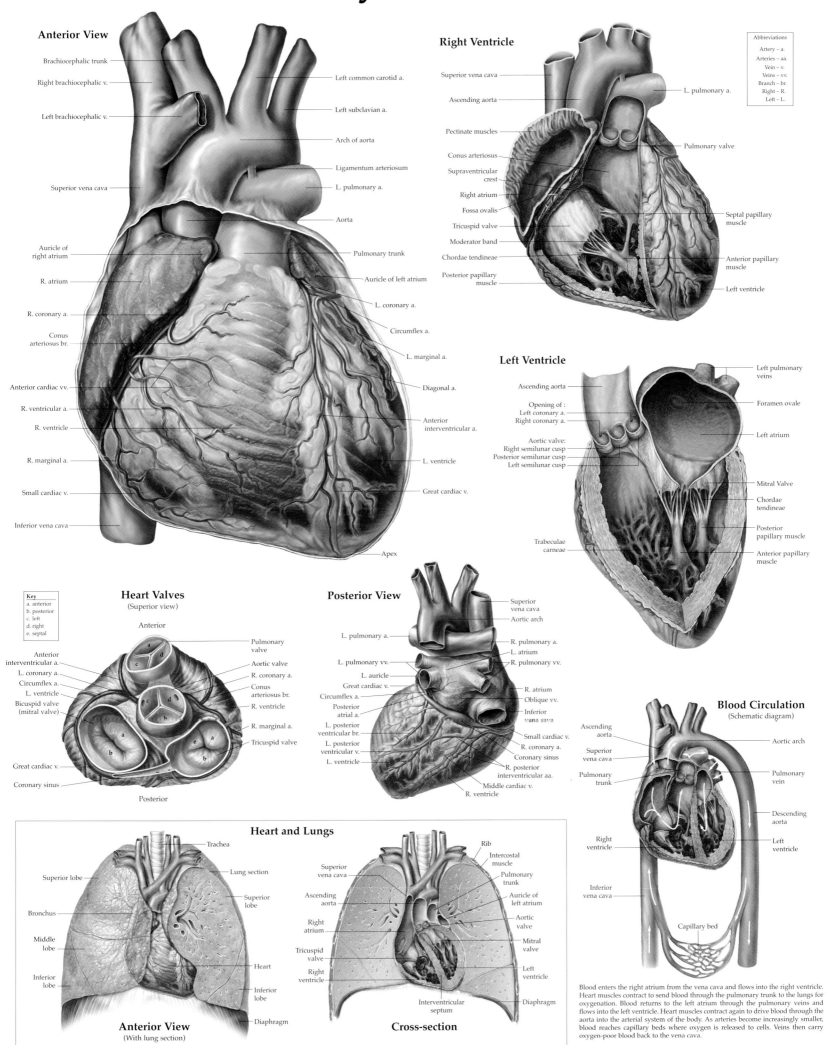

Anterior View

- Brachiocephalic trunk
- Right brachiocephalic v.
- Left brachiocephalic v.
- Superior vena cava
- Auricle of right atrium
- R. atrium
- R. coronary a.
- Conus arteriosus br.
- Anterior cardiac vv.
- R. ventricular a.
- R. ventricle
- R. marginal a.
- Small cardiac v.
- Inferior vena cava
- Left common carotid a.
- Left subclavian a.
- Arch of aorta
- Ligamentum arteriosum
- L. pulmonary a.
- Aorta
- Pulmonary trunk
- Auricle of left atrium
- L. coronary a.
- Circumflex a.
- L. marginal a.
- Diagonal a.
- Anterior interventricular a.
- L. ventricle
- Great cardiac v.
- Apex

Right Ventricle

Abbreviations
Artery – a.
Arteries – aa.
Vein – v.
Veins – vv.
Branch – br.
Right – R.
Left – L.

- Superior vena cava
- Ascending aorta
- Pectinate muscles
- Conus arteriosus
- Supraventricular crest
- Right atrium
- Fossa ovalis
- Tricuspid valve
- Moderator band
- Chordae tendineae
- Posterior papillary muscle
- L. pulmonary a.
- Pulmonary valve
- Septal papillary muscle
- Anterior papillary muscle
- Left ventricle

Left Ventricle

- Ascending aorta
- Opening of :
  Left coronary a.
  Right coronary a.
- Aortic valve:
  Right semilunar cusp
  Posterior semilunar cusp
  Left semilunar cusp
- Trabeculae carneae
- Left pulmonary veins
- Foramen ovale
- Left atrium
- Mitral Valve
- Chordae tendineae
- Posterior papillary muscle
- Anterior papillary muscle

Heart Valves
(Superior view)

Key
a. anterior
b. posterior
c. left
d. right
e. septal

Anterior

- Anterior interventricular a.
- L. coronary a.
- Circumflex a.
- L. ventricle
- Bicuspid valve (mitral valve)
- Great cardiac v.
- Coronary sinus
- Pulmonary valve
- Aortic valve
- R. coronary a.
- Conus arteriosus br.
- R. ventricle
- R. marginal a.
- Tricuspid valve

Posterior

Posterior View

- L. pulmonary a.
- L. pulmonary vv.
- L. auricle
- Great cardiac v.
- Circumflex a.
- Posterior atrial a.
- L. posterior ventricular br.
- L. posterior ventricular v.
- L. ventricle
- Superior vena cava
- Aortic arch
- R. pulmonary a.
- L. atrium
- R. pulmonary vv.
- R. atrium
- Oblique vv.
- Inferior vena cava
- Small cardiac v.
- R. coronary a.
- Coronary sinus
- R. posterior interventricular aa.
- Middle cardiac v.
- R. ventricle

Blood Circulation
(Schematic diagram)

- Ascending aorta
- Superior vena cava
- Pulmonary trunk
- Right ventricle
- Inferior vena cava
- Aortic arch
- Pulmonary vein
- Descending aorta
- Left ventricle
- Capillary bed

Heart and Lungs

Anterior View
(With lung section)

- Trachea
- Lung section
- Superior lobe
- Bronchus
- Middle lobe
- Inferior lobe
- Heart
- Inferior lobe
- Diaphragm

Cross-section

- Superior vena cava
- Ascending aorta
- Right atrium
- Tricuspid valve
- Right ventricle
- Rib
- Intercostal muscle
- Pulmonary trunk
- Auricle of left atrium
- Aortic valve
- Mitral valve
- Left ventricle
- Interventricular septum
- Diaphragm

Blood enters the right atrium from the vena cava and flows into the right ventricle. Heart muscles contract to send blood through the pulmonary trunk to the lungs for oxygenation. Blood returns to the left atrium through the pulmonary veins and flows into the left ventricle. Heart muscles contract again to drive blood through the aorta into the arterial system of the body. As arteries become increasingly smaller, blood reaches capillary beds where oxygen is released to cells. Veins then carry oxygen-poor blood back to the vena cava.

©2014 Wolters Kluwer

Hip and Knee

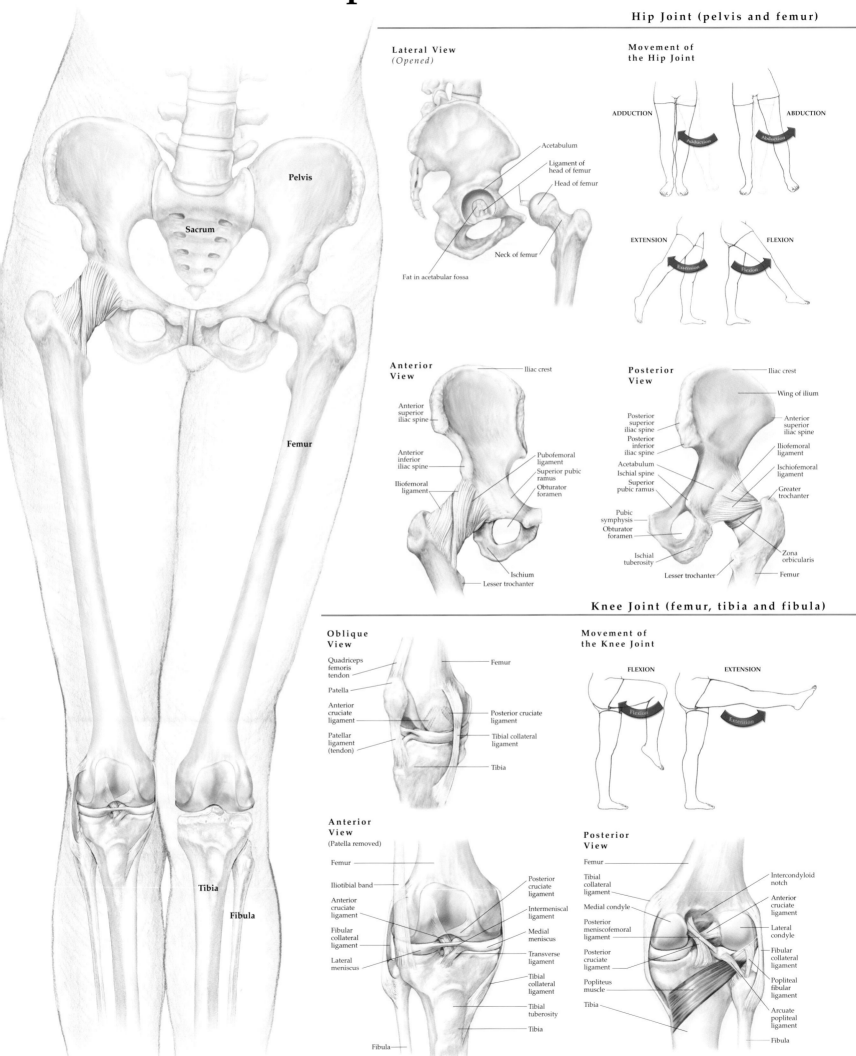

Hip Joint (pelvis and femur)

Lateral View *(Opened)*

Acetabulum
Ligament of head of femur
Head of femur
Neck of femur
Fat in acetabular fossa

Movement of the Hip Joint

ADDUCTION — Adduction
ABDUCTION — Abduction
EXTENSION — Extension
FLEXION — Flexion

Anterior View

Iliac crest
Anterior superior iliac spine
Anterior inferior iliac spine
Iliofemoral ligament
Pubofemoral ligament
Superior pubic ramus
Obturator foramen
Ischium
Lesser trochanter

Posterior View

Iliac crest
Wing of ilium
Posterior superior iliac spine
Posterior inferior iliac spine
Acetabulum
Ischial spine
Superior pubic ramus
Pubic symphysis
Obturator foramen
Ischial tuberosity
Lesser trochanter
Anterior superior iliac spine
Iliofemoral ligament
Ischiofemoral ligament
Greater trochanter
Zona orbicularis
Femur

Knee Joint (femur, tibia and fibula)

Oblique View

Quadriceps femoris tendon
Patella
Anterior cruciate ligament
Patellar ligament (tendon)
Femur
Posterior cruciate ligament
Tibial collateral ligament
Tibia

Movement of the Knee Joint

FLEXION — Flexion
EXTENSION — Extension

Anterior View (Patella removed)

Femur
Iliotibial band
Anterior cruciate ligament
Fibular collateral ligament
Lateral meniscus
Posterior cruciate ligament
Intermeniscal ligament
Medial meniscus
Transverse ligament
Tibial collateral ligament
Tibial tuberosity
Tibia
Fibula

Posterior View

Femur
Tibial collateral ligament
Medial condyle
Posterior meniscofemoral ligament
Posterior cruciate ligament
Popliteus muscle
Tibia
Intercondyloid notch
Anterior cruciate ligament
Lateral condyle
Fibular collateral ligament
Popliteal fibular ligament
Arcuate popliteal ligament
Fibula

Pelvis
Sacrum
Femur
Tibia
Fibula

©2014 Wolters Kluwer

Ligaments of the Joints

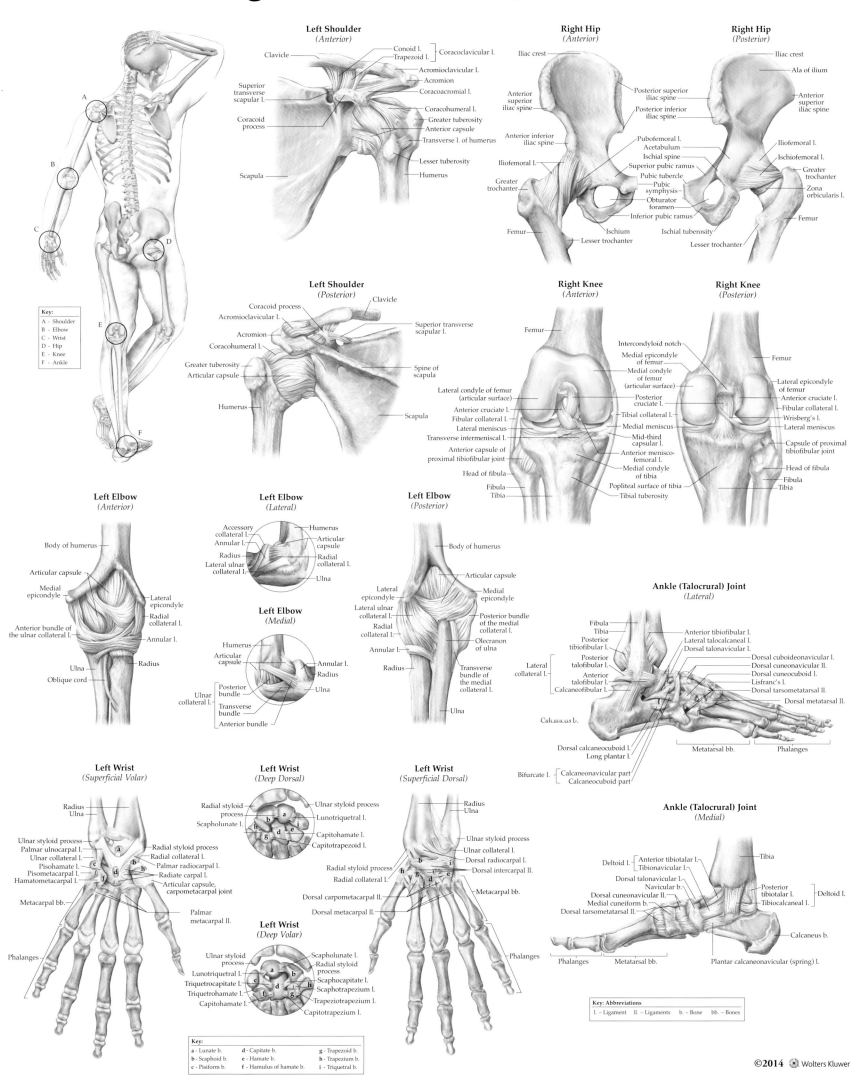

Left Shoulder *(Anterior)*

Clavicle — Conoid l. / Trapezoid l. — Coracoclavicular l.
Acromioclavicular l.
Acromion
Superior transverse scapular l.
Coracoacromial l.
Coracohumeral l.
Coracoid process
Greater tuberosity
Anterior capsule
Transverse l. of humerus
Lesser tuberosity
Scapula
Humerus

Right Hip *(Anterior)*

Iliac crest
Anterior superior iliac spine
Posterior superior iliac spine
Posterior inferior iliac spine
Anterior inferior iliac spine
Pubofemoral l.
Acetabulum
Iliofemoral l.
Ischial spine
Superior pubic ramus
Greater trochanter
Pubic tubercle
Pubic symphysis
Obturator foramen
Inferior pubic ramus
Femur
Ischium
Lesser trochanter

Right Hip *(Posterior)*

Iliac crest
Ala of ilium
Anterior superior iliac spine
Iliofemoral l.
Ischiofemoral l.
Greater trochanter
Zona orbicularis l.
Femur
Ischial tuberosity
Lesser trochanter

Left Shoulder *(Posterior)*

Coracoid process
Clavicle
Acromioclavicular l.
Superior transverse scapular l.
Acromion
Coracohumeral l.
Greater tuberosity
Articular capsule
Spine of scapula
Humerus
Scapula

Right Knee *(Anterior)*

Femur
Intercondyloid notch
Medial epicondyle of femur
Medial condyle of femur (articular surface)
Lateral condyle of femur (articular surface)
Posterior cruciate l.
Anterior cruciate l.
Tibial collateral l.
Fibular collateral l.
Medial meniscus
Lateral meniscus
Transverse intermeniscal l.
Mid-third capsular l.
Anterior capsule of proximal tibiofibular joint
Anterior menisco-femoral l.
Medial condyle of tibia
Head of fibula
Popliteal surface of tibia
Fibula
Tibial tuberosity
Tibia

Right Knee *(Posterior)*

Femur
Lateral epicondyle of femur
Anterior cruciate l.
Fibular collateral l.
Wrisberg's l.
Lateral meniscus
Capsule of proximal tibiofibular joint
Head of fibula
Fibula
Tibia

Left Elbow *(Anterior)*

Body of humerus
Articular capsule
Medial epicondyle
Lateral epicondyle
Radial collateral l.
Anterior bundle of the ulnar collateral l.
Annular l.
Ulna
Radius
Oblique cord

Left Elbow *(Lateral)*

Accessory collateral l.
Humerus
Annular l.
Articular capsule
Radius
Radial collateral l.
Lateral ulnar collateral l.
Ulna

Left Elbow *(Medial)*

Humerus
Articular capsule
Annular l.
Radius
Ulna
Ulnar collateral l.
Posterior bundle
Transverse bundle
Anterior bundle

Left Elbow *(Posterior)*

Body of humerus
Articular capsule
Lateral epicondyle
Medial epicondyle
Lateral ulnar collateral l.
Radial collateral l.
Posterior bundle of the medial collateral l.
Annular l.
Olecranon of ulna
Radius
Transverse bundle of the medial collateral l.
Ulna

Ankle (Talocrural) Joint *(Lateral)*

Fibula
Tibia
Posterior tibiofibular l.
Anterior tibiofibular l.
Lateral talocalcaneal l.
Dorsal talonavicular l.
Posterior talofibular l.
Lateral collateral l.
Anterior talofibular l.
Calcaneofibular l.
Dorsal cuboideonavicular l.
Dorsal cuneonavicular ll.
Dorsal cuneocuboid l.
Lisfranc's l.
Dorsal tarsometatarsal ll.
Dorsal metatarsal ll.
Calcaneus b.
Dorsal calcaneocuboid l.
Long plantar l.
Metatarsal bb.
Phalanges
Bifurcate l.
Calcaneonavicular part
Calcaneocuboid part

Left Wrist *(Superficial Volar)*

Radius
Ulna
Ulnar styloid process
Palmar ulnocarpal l.
Ulnar collateral l.
Pisohamate l.
Pisometacarpal l.
Hamatometacarpal l.
Metacarpal bb.
Radial styloid process
Radial collateral l.
Palmar radiocarpal l.
Radiate carpal l.
Articular capsule, carpometacarpal joint
Palmar metacarpal ll.
Phalanges

Left Wrist *(Deep Dorsal)*

Radial styloid process
Scapholunate l.
Ulnar styloid process
Lunotriquetral l.
Capitohamate l.
Capitotrapezoid l.

a, b, c, d, e, f, g, h, i

Left Wrist *(Superficial Dorsal)*

Radius
Ulna
Ulnar styloid process
Ulnar collateral l.
Dorsal radiocarpal l.
Dorsal intercarpal ll.
Radial styloid process
Radial collateral l.
Dorsal carpometacarpal ll.
Dorsal metacarpal ll.
Metacarpal bb.
Phalanges

Left Wrist *(Deep Volar)*

Ulnar styloid process
Scapholunate l.
Lunotriquetral l.
Radial styloid process
Triquetrocapitate l.
Scaphocapitate l.
Triquetrohamate l.
Scaphotrapezium l.
Capitohamate l.
Trapeziotrapezium l.
Capitotrapezium l.

a, b, c, d, e, f, g, h

Ankle (Talocrural) Joint *(Medial)*

Deltoid l.
Anterior tibiotalar l.
Tibionavicular l.
Tibia
Dorsal talonavicular l.
Navicular b.
Posterior tibiotalar l.
Dorsal cuneonavicular ll.
Medial cuneiform b.
Tibiocalcaneal l.
Deltoid l.
Dorsal tarsometatarsal ll.
Calcaneus b.
Phalanges
Metatarsal bb.
Plantar calcaneonavicular (spring) l.

Key:
A - Shoulder
B - Elbow
C - Wrist
D - Hip
E - Knee
F - Ankle

Key:
a - Lunate b.
b - Scaphoid b.
c - Pisiform b.
d - Capitate b.
e - Hamate b.
f - Hamulus of hamate b.
g - Trapezoid b.
h - Trapezium b.
i - Triquetral b.

Key: Abbreviations
l. – Ligament   ll. – Ligaments   b. – Bone   bb. – Bones

©2014 Wolters Kluwer

Pregnancy and Birth

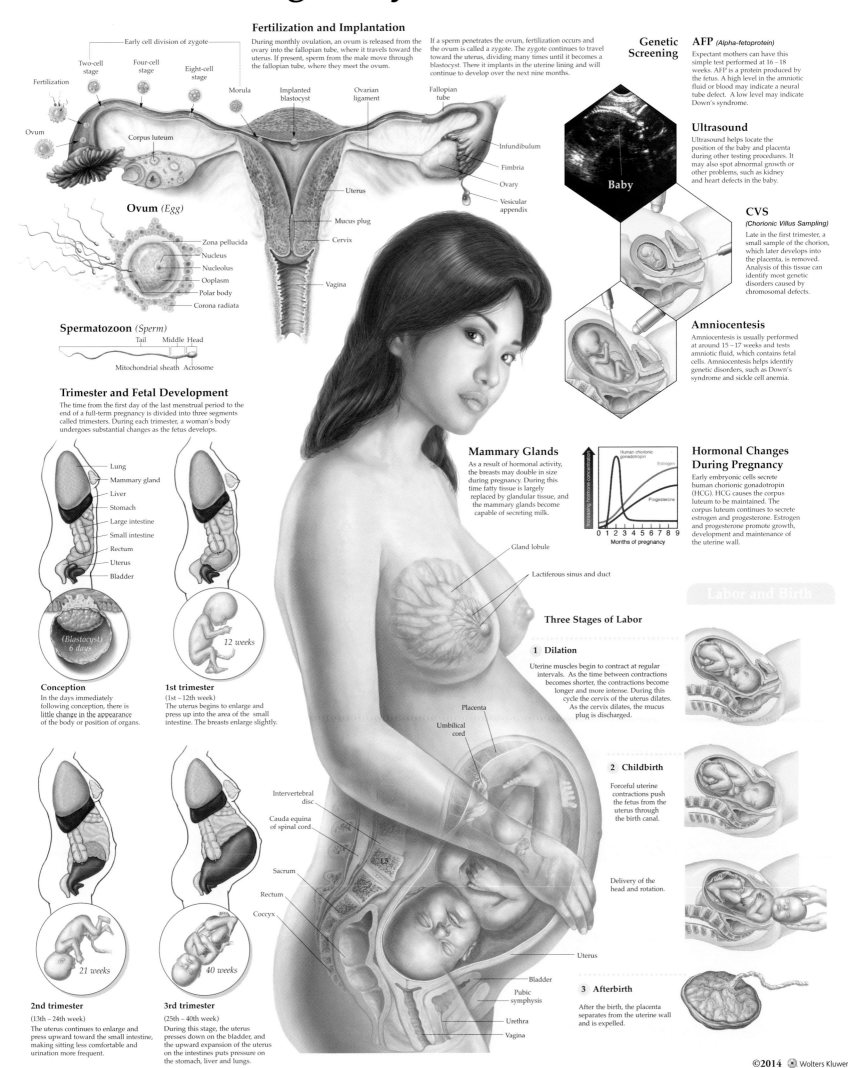

Fertilization and Implantation

Early cell division of zygote

Two-cell stage
Four-cell stage
Eight-cell stage
Fertilization
Morula
Ovum
Corpus luteum
Implanted blastocyst
Ovarian ligament
Fallopian tube
Infundibulum
Fimbria
Ovary
Uterus
Vesicular appendix
Mucus plug
Cervix
Vagina

During monthly ovulation, an ovum is released from the ovary into the fallopian tube, where it travels toward the uterus. If present, sperm from the male move through the fallopian tube, where they meet the ovum.

If a sperm penetrates the ovum, fertilization occurs and the ovum is called a zygote. The zygote continues to travel toward the uterus, dividing many times until it becomes a blastocyst. There it implants in the uterine lining and will continue to develop over the next nine months.

Ovum (Egg)

Zona pellucida
Nucleus
Nucleolus
Ooplasm
Polar body
Corona radiata

Spermatozoon (Sperm)

Tail
Middle
Head
Mitochondrial sheath
Acrosome

Trimester and Fetal Development

The time from the first day of the last menstrual period to the end of a full-term pregnancy is divided into three segments called trimesters. During each trimester, a woman's body undergoes substantial changes as the fetus develops.

Lung
Mammary gland
Liver
Stomach
Large intestine
Small intestine
Rectum
Uterus
Bladder

(Blastocyst) 6 days

12 weeks

Conception
In the days immediately following conception, there is little change in the appearance of the body or position of organs.

1st trimester
(1st – 12th week)
The uterus begins to enlarge and press up into the area of the small intestine. The breasts enlarge slightly.

21 weeks

40 weeks

2nd trimester
(13th – 24th week)
The uterus continues to enlarge and press upward toward the small intestine, making sitting less comfortable and urination more frequent.

3rd trimester
(25th – 40th week)
During this stage, the uterus presses down on the bladder, and the upward expansion of the uterus on the intestines puts pressure on the stomach, liver and lungs.

Genetic Screening

AFP (Alpha-fetoprotein)
Expectant mothers can have this simple test performed at 16 – 18 weeks. AFP is a protein produced by the fetus. A high level in the amniotic fluid or blood may indicate a neural tube defect. A low level may indicate Down's syndrome.

Baby

Ultrasound
Ultrasound helps locate the position of the baby and placenta during other testing procedures. It may also spot abnormal growth or other problems, such as kidney and heart defects in the baby.

CVS
(Chorionic Villus Sampling)
Late in the first trimester, a small sample of the chorion, which later develops into the placenta, is removed. Analysis of this tissue can identify most genetic disorders caused by chromosomal defects.

Amniocentesis
Amniocentesis is usually performed at around 15 – 17 weeks and tests amniotic fluid, which contains fetal cells. Amniocentesis helps identify genetic disorders, such as Down's syndrome and sickle cell anemia.

Mammary Glands
As a result of hormonal activity, the breasts may double in size during pregnancy. During this time fatty tissue is largely replaced by glandular tissue, and the mammary glands become capable of secreting milk.

Gland lobule
Lactiferous sinus and duct

Hormonal Changes During Pregnancy
Early embryonic cells secrete human chorionic gonadotropin (HCG). HCG causes the corpus luteum to be maintained. The corpus luteum continues to secrete estrogen and progesterone. Estrogen and progesterone promote growth, development and maintenance of the uterine wall.

Human chorionic gonadotropin
Estrogen
Progesterone
Increasing hormone concentration
0 1 2 3 4 5 6 7 8 9
Months of pregnancy

Labor and Birth

Three Stages of Labor

1 Dilation
Uterine muscles begin to contract at regular intervals. As the time between contractions becomes shorter, the contractions become longer and more intense. During this cycle the cervix of the uterus dilates. As the cervix dilates, the mucus plug is discharged.

2 Childbirth
Forceful uterine contractions push the fetus from the uterus through the birth canal.

Delivery of the head and rotation.

Placenta
Umbilical cord
Intervertebral disc
Cauda equina of spinal cord
Sacrum
Rectum
Coccyx
L5
Uterus
Bladder
Pubic symphysis
Urethra
Vagina

3 Afterbirth
After the birth, the placenta separates from the uterine wall and is expelled.

©2014 Wolters Kluwer

The Prostate

Hormonal Influence on the Prostate

The prostate functions continuously, producing fluid which empties into the urethra. Hormones from the **pituitary gland** direct the **adrenal glands** and the **testes** to send chemical signals to the **prostate** to promote fluid production.

Pituitary
Adrenal gland
Kidney
Ureter
Urinary bladder
Prostate
Testis

What is the Prostate?

The prostate is a gland consisting of fibrous, muscular and glandular tissue surrounding the urethra below the urinary bladder. Its function is to secrete prostatic fluid as a medium for semen, helping it to reach the female reproductive tract. Within the prostate, the urethra is joined by two ejaculatory ducts. During sexual activity, the prostate acts as a valve between the urinary and reproductive tracts. This enables semen to ejaculate without mixing with urine. Prostatic fluid is delivered by the contraction of muscles around gland tissue. Nerve and hormonal influences control the secretory and muscular functions of the prostate.

Normal Prostate (sagittal section)

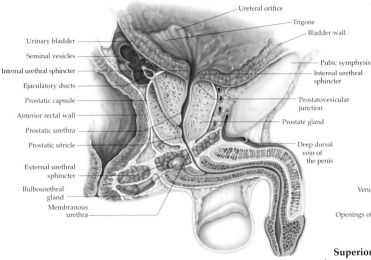

Ureteral orifice
Trigone
Bladder wall
Urinary bladder
Seminal vesicles
Internal urethral sphincter
Ejaculatory ducts
Prostatic capsule
Anterior rectal wall
Prostatic urethra
Prostatic utricle
External urethral sphincter
Bulbourethral gland
Membranous urethra
Pubic symphysis
Internal urethral sphincter
Prostatovesicular junction
Prostate gland
Deep dorsal vein of the penis

Posterior View (dissected)

Fibromuscular wall of bladder
Ductus deferens
Ureter
Ampulla of ductus deferens
Seminal vesicles
Levator ani m.
Prostatic utricle
Peritoneal covering over bladder dome
Membranous urethra

Anterior View with Exposed Prostatic Urethra

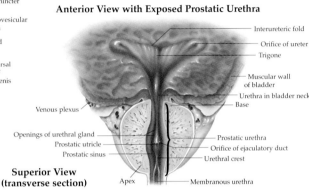

Interureteric fold
Orifice of ureter
Trigone
Muscular wall of bladder
Urethra in bladder neck
Base
Venous plexus
Openings of urethral gland
Prostatic utricle
Prostatic sinus
Apex
Prostatic urethra
Orifice of ejaculatory duct
Urethral crest
Membranous urethra

Superior View (transverse section)

Prostate glandular tissue lobes
Prostatic urethra
Prostatic utricle
Ejaculatory ducts

Secretory gland with grape-shaped **acinus** end.

Vasculature and Innervation

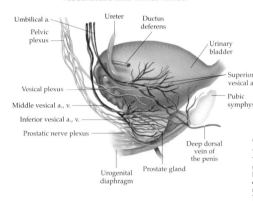

Umbilical a.
Pelvic plexus
Ureter
Ductus deferens
Urinary bladder
Superior vesical a., v.
Vesical plexus
Middle vesical a., v.
Inferior vesical a., v.
Prostatic nerve plexus
Urogenital diaphragm
Prostate gland
Pubic symphysis
Deep dorsal vein of the penis

Zones of the Prostate

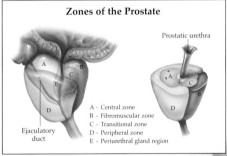

Prostatic urethra
Ejaculatory duct

A - Central zone
B - Fibromuscular zone
C - Transitional zone
D - Peripheral zone
E - Periurethral gland region

Glands of the Prostate

The prostate is mainly filled with secretory glands. These glands are made of many ducts with grape-shaped saccule ends or "acini". Secretory cells lining the ducts are stimulated by hormones to expel prostatic fluid. During sexual activity muscle contracts and secrete prostatic fluid. The basal cell, also found lining the ducts of the prostate, may be responsible for most types of prostatic hyperplasia as a result of uncontrolled prostatic tissue growth.

Prostatic duct

Secretory cells are the most numerous in the gland and form the inner lining.

The **basal cell** is located below the lining surface and may function to rebuild prostatic tissue after infection or other damage.

Fibromuscular stroma
Ductal lumen
Prostatic fluid

Benign Prostatic Hyperplasia (BPH)

Benign Prostatic Hyperplasia (BPH), is the most common type of tumor in mature men. It is a benign growth, which means it may enlarge but will not spread to other locations in the body. The tumor can cause discomfort and may grow to completely close the bladder neck, preventing urination. This condition occurs because the tumor usually grows in the transitional zone and periurethral gland region located at the prostate base near the bladder neck.

Early BPH:

Narrowing of the prostatic urethra causing difficulty in starting, maintaining, and stopping urination.

Prostatic urethra

Prostatitis

Prostatitis is an uncomfortable condition in which the prostate becomes inflamed and swollen due to an infection. Prostatitis can make urinating painful.

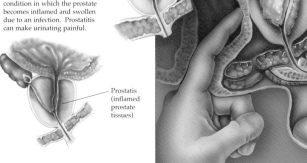

Prostatis (inflamed prostate tissues)

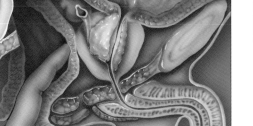

A **digital rectal exam** is very useful in detecting early signs of prostatic enlargement.

Prostate Cancer

Prostate carcinoma is the most common malignant tumor in men. Unlike BPH, prostate cancer not only enlarges but also metastasizes (spreads) to other parts of the body through lymphatic and venous channels.

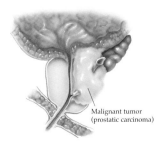

Malignant tumor (prostatic carcinoma)

Pathways of Prostate Cancer Spread

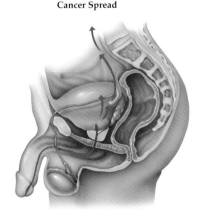

©2014 Wolters Kluwer

Shoulder and Elbow

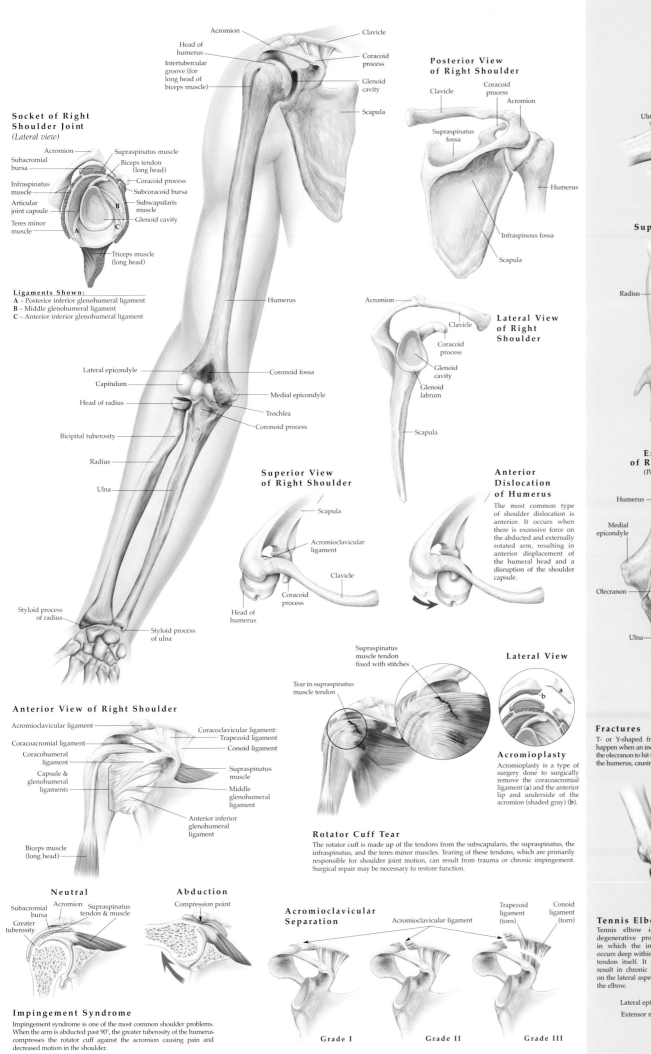

Socket of Right Shoulder Joint
(Lateral view)

Acromion
Subacromial bursa
Supraspinatus muscle
Biceps tendon (long head)
Infraspinatus muscle
Coracoid process
Articular joint capsule
Subcoracoid bursa
Subscapularis muscle
Teres minor muscle
Glenoid cavity
Triceps muscle (long head)

Ligaments Shown:
A – Posterior inferior glenohumeral ligament
B – Middle glenohumeral ligament
C – Anterior inferior glenohumeral ligament

Acromion
Head of humerus
Clavicle
Intertubercular groove (for long head of biceps muscle)
Coracoid process
Glenoid cavity
Scapula

Humerus

Lateral epicondyle
Capitulum
Head of radius
Coronoid fossa
Medial epicondyle
Trochlea
Coronoid process
Bicipital tuberosity
Radius
Ulna

Styloid process of radius
Styloid process of ulna

Posterior View of Right Shoulder

Clavicle
Coracoid process
Acromion
Supraspinatus fossa
Humerus
Infraspinous fossa
Scapula

Lateral View of Right Shoulder

Acromion
Clavicle
Coracoid process
Glenoid cavity
Glenoid labrum
Scapula

Superior View of Right Shoulder

Scapula
Acromioclavicular ligament
Clavicle
Coracoid process
Head of humerus

Anterior Dislocation of Humerus

The most common type of shoulder dislocation is anterior. It occurs when there is excessive force on the abducted and externally rotated arm, resulting in anterior displacement of the humeral head and a disruption of the shoulder capsule.

Anterior View of Right Shoulder

Acromioclavicular ligament
Coracoacromial ligament
Coracohumeral ligament
Capsule & glenohumeral ligaments
Coracoclavicular ligament: Trapezoid ligament
Conoid ligament
Supraspinatus muscle
Middle glenohumeral ligament
Anterior inferior glenohumeral ligament
Biceps muscle (long head)

Impingement Syndrome

Impingement syndrome is one of the most common shoulder problems. When the arm is abducted past 90°, the greater tuberosity of the humerus compresses the rotator cuff against the acromion causing pain and decreased motion in the shoulder.

Neutral
Subacromial bursa
Acromion
Supraspinatus tendon & muscle
Greater tuberosity

Abduction
Compression point

Acromioclavicular Separation

Acromioclavicular ligament
Trapezoid ligament (torn)
Conoid ligament (torn)

Grade I
Grade II
Grade III

Supraspinatus muscle tendon fixed with stitches
Tear in supraspinatus muscle tendon

Lateral View

a
b

Acromioplasty

Acromioplasty is a type of surgery done to surgically remove the coracoacromial ligament (a) and the anterior lip and underside of the acromion (shaded gray) (b).

Rotator Cuff Tear

The rotator cuff is made up of the tendons from the subscapularis, the supraspinatus, the infraspinatus, and the teres minor muscles. Tearing of these tendons, which are primarily responsible for shoulder joint motion, can result from trauma or chronic impingement. Surgical repair may be necessary to restore function.

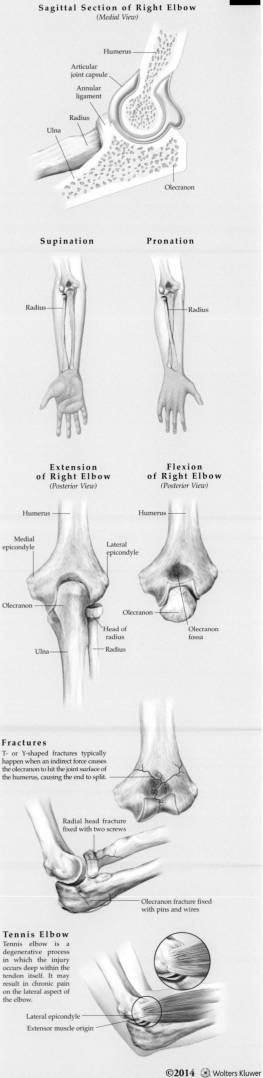

Sagittal Section of Right Elbow
(Medial View)

Humerus
Articular joint capsule
Annular ligament
Radius
Ulna
Olecranon

Supination
Radius

Pronation
Radius

Extension of Right Elbow
(Posterior View)

Humerus
Medial epicondyle
Olecranon
Head of radius
Ulna
Radius

Flexion of Right Elbow
(Posterior View)

Humerus
Lateral epicondyle
Olecranon
Olecranon fossa

Fractures

T- or Y-shaped fractures typically happen when an indirect force causes the olecranon to hit the joint surface of the humerus, causing the end to split.

Radial head fracture fixed with two screws
Olecranon fracture fixed with pins and wires

Tennis Elbow

Tennis elbow is a degenerative process in which the injury occurs deep within the tendon itself. It may result in chronic pain on the lateral aspect of the elbow.

Lateral epicondyle
Extensor muscle origin

©2014 Wolters Kluwer

The Skin and Common Disorders

Normal Anatomy

The skin is the body's largest organ. It covers the entire body and weighs approximately six pounds. The skin includes two primary layers: the outer epidermis and the inner dermis. The epidermis has important protective functions. It protects against injury and excessive water loss. It also prevents disease-causing microorganisms from entering the body.

The thick dermis contains blood vessels, nerve endings, and glands that respond to heat, pressure, and pain. Beneath the dermis, the subcutaneous layer is made up of loose connective tissue and fat (adipose) tissue. This layer acts as a cushion for the skin, helps maintain body heat, and is a store of energy.

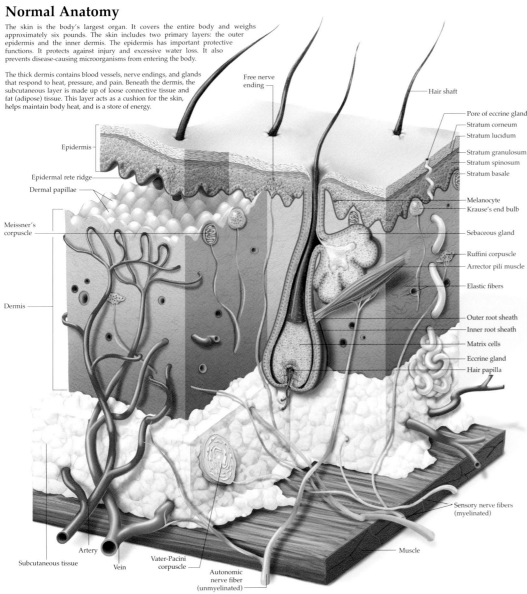

Epidermis

Epidermal rete ridge

Dermal papillae

Meissner's corpuscle

Dermis

Subcutaneous tissue

Artery

Vein

Vater-Pacini corpuscle

Autonomic nerve fiber (unmyelinated)

Free nerve ending

Hair shaft

Pore of eccrine gland
Stratum corneum
Stratum lucidum
Stratum granulosum
Stratum spinosum
Stratum basale

Melanocyte
Krause's end bulb

Sebaceous gland

Ruffini corpuscle
Arrector pili muscle

Elastic fibers

Outer root sheath
Inner root sheath
Matrix cells
Eccrine gland
Hair papilla

Sensory nerve fibers (myelinated)

Muscle

Derivatives of Skin

Derivatives of skin include hair, sebaceous glands, sweat glands and nails. These structures all derive from specialized areas of the epidermis that grow down into the dermis.

Hair

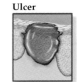

Inner root sheath
Huxley's layer
Henle's layer

Medulla
Cortex
Cuticle

Hair shaft

Outer root sheath
Glassy membrane
Connective tissue sheath

Nail

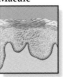

Lateral nail fold
Nail plate
Nail bed

Hyponychium
Lunula
Eponychium
Nail matrix
Nail root

Types of Skin Lesions

Fissure
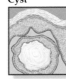
A painful, cracklike lesion of the skin that extends at least into the dermis.

Ulcer

A craterlike lesion of the skin that usually extends at least into the dermis.

Cyst
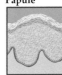
A closed sac in or under the skin that contains fluid or semisolid material.

Macule

A small, discolored spot or patch on the skin.

Papule
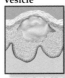
A solid, raised lesion that is usually less than 1 cm in diameter.

Wheal

A raised reddish area, often itchy, lasting 24 hours or less.

Vesicle
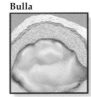
A small fluid filled blister, usually 1 cm or less in diameter.

Pustule

A small, pus filled lesion. If it contains a hair it is called a follicular pustule.

Bulla
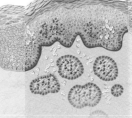
A large fluid filled blister, usually 1 cm or more in diameter.

Nodule

A raised lesion detectable by touch, usually 1 cm or more in diameter.

Common Skin Disorders

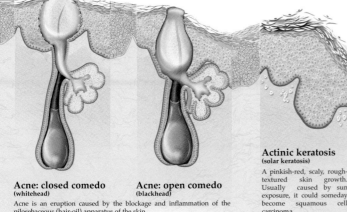

Acne: closed comedo (whitehead)

Acne: open comedo (blackhead)

Acne is an eruption caused by the blockage and inflammation of the pilosebaceous (hair-oil) apparatus of the skin.

Actinic keratosis (solar keratosis)
A pinkish-red, scaly, rough-textured skin growth. Usually caused by sun exposure, it could someday become squamous cell carcinoma.

Junctional nevus (mole)
A flat or slightly raised growth that can be rough or smooth and varies in color from light to dark brown.

Urticaria (hives)
Areas of itchy wheals that occur as the result of an allergic reaction.

Squamous cell carcinoma
A slow-growing, malignant tumor of the skin that usually affects areas that have been exposed to the sun. If not treated, it can spread to other parts of the body.

Verruca vulgaris (wart)
A common, noncancerous viral infection of the skin and nearby mucous membranes.

Seborrheic keratosis (basal cell papilloma)
A harmless, wartlike growth that is usually brown or black in color.

Dermatofibroma (fibrous histiocytoma, sclerosing hemangioma)
A noncancerous skin tumor that has become hardened, cellular, and fibrous.

Basal cell carcinoma
The most common type of skin cancer. Beginning as a papule, it enlarges, eventually developing a central crater. It usually only spreads locally.

©2014 Wolters Kluwer

The Human Skull

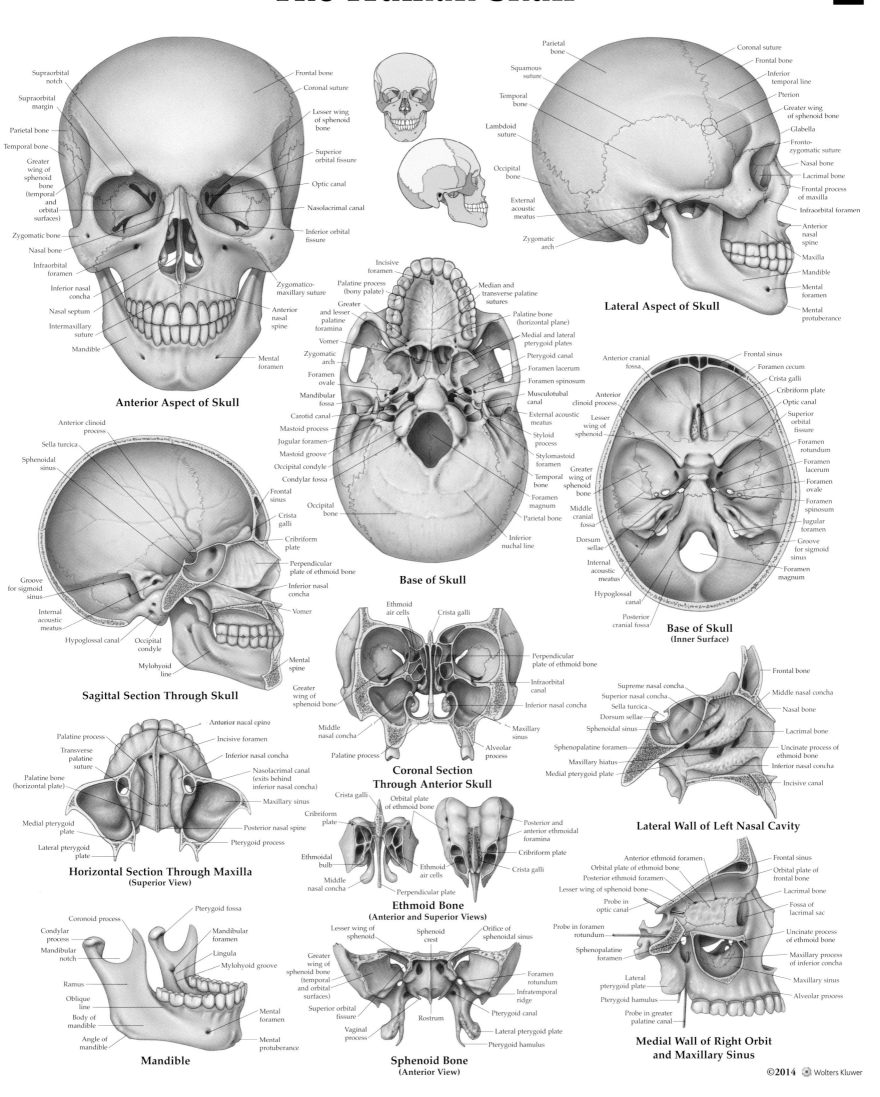

Anterior Aspect of Skull

Supraorbital notch
Supraorbital margin
Parietal bone
Temporal bone
Greater wing of sphenoid bone (temporal and orbital surfaces)
Zygomatic bone
Nasal bone
Infraorbital foramen
Inferior nasal concha
Nasal septum
Intermaxillary suture
Mandible
Frontal bone
Coronal suture
Lesser wing of sphenoid bone
Superior orbital fissure
Optic canal
Nasolacrimal canal
Inferior orbital fissure
Zygomatico-maxillary suture
Anterior nasal spine
Mental foramen

Lateral Aspect of Skull

Parietal bone
Squamous suture
Temporal bone
Lambdoid suture
Occipital bone
External acoustic meatus
Zygomatic arch
Coronal suture
Frontal bone
Inferior temporal line
Pterion
Greater wing of sphenoid bone
Glabella
Fronto-zygomatic suture
Nasal bone
Lacrimal bone
Frontal process of maxilla
Infraorbital foramen
Anterior nasal spine
Maxilla
Mandible
Mental foramen
Mental protuberance

Base of Skull

Incisive foramen
Palatine process (bony palate)
Greater and lesser palatine foramina
Vomer
Zygomatic arch
Foramen ovale
Mandibular fossa
Carotid canal
Mastoid process
Jugular foramen
Mastoid groove
Occipital condyle
Condylar fossa
Occipital bone
Median and transverse palatine sutures
Palatine bone (horizontal plane)
Medial and lateral pterygoid plates
Pterygoid canal
Foramen lacerum
Foramen spinosum
Musculotubal canal
External acoustic meatus
Styloid process
Stylomastoid foramen
Temporal bone
Foramen magnum
Parietal bone
Inferior nuchal line

Base of Skull (Inner Surface)

Anterior cranial fossa
Anterior clinoid process
Lesser wing of sphenoid
Greater wing of sphenoid bone
Middle cranial fossa
Dorsum sellae
Internal acoustic meatus
Hypoglossal canal
Posterior cranial fossa
Frontal sinus
Foramen cecum
Crista galli
Cribriform plate
Optic canal
Superior orbital fissure
Foramen rotundum
Foramen lacerum
Foramen ovale
Foramen spinosum
Jugular foramen
Groove for sigmoid sinus
Foramen magnum

Sagittal Section Through Skull

Anterior clinoid process
Sella turcica
Sphenoidal sinus
Groove for sigmoid sinus
Internal acoustic meatus
Hypoglossal canal
Occipital condyle
Mylohyoid line
Frontal sinus
Crista galli
Cribriform plate
Perpendicular plate of ethmoid bone
Inferior nasal concha
Vomer
Mental spine

Coronal Section Through Anterior Skull

Ethmoid air cells
Crista galli
Greater wing of sphenoid bone
Middle nasal concha
Palatine process
Perpendicular plate of ethmoid bone
Infraorbital canal
Inferior nasal concha
Maxillary sinus
Alveolar process

Horizontal Section Through Maxilla (Superior View)

Palatine process
Transverse palatine suture
Palatine bone (horizontal plate)
Medial pterygoid plate
Lateral pterygoid plate
Anterior nasal spine
Incisive foramen
Inferior nasal concha
Nasolacrimal canal (exits behind inferior nasal concha)
Maxillary sinus
Posterior nasal spine
Pterygoid process

Ethmoid Bone (Anterior and Superior Views)

Crista galli
Cribriform plate
Ethmoidal bulb
Middle nasal concha
Orbital plate of ethmoid bone
Posterior and anterior ethmoidal foramina
Cribriform plate
Crista galli
Ethmoid air cells
Perpendicular plate

Lateral Wall of Left Nasal Cavity

Supreme nasal concha
Superior nasal concha
Sella turcica
Dorsum sellae
Sphenoidal sinus
Sphenopalatine foramen
Maxillary hiatus
Medial pterygoid plate
Frontal bone
Middle nasal concha
Nasal bone
Lacrimal bone
Uncinate process of ethmoid bone
Inferior nasal concha
Incisive canal

Mandible

Coronoid process
Condylar process
Mandibular notch
Ramus
Oblique line
Body of mandible
Angle of mandible
Pterygoid fossa
Mandibular foramen
Lingula
Mylohyoid groove
Mental foramen
Mental protuberance

Sphenoid Bone (Anterior View)

Lesser wing of sphenoid
Greater wing of sphenoid bone (temporal and orbital surfaces)
Superior orbital fissure
Vaginal process
Sphenoid crest
Orifice of sphenoidal sinus
Foramen rotundum
Infratemporal ridge
Pterygoid canal
Lateral pterygoid plate
Pterygoid hamulus
Rostrum

Medial Wall of Right Orbit and Maxillary Sinus

Anterior ethmoid foramen
Orbital plate of ethmoid bone
Posterior ethmoid foramen
Lesser wing of sphenoid bone
Probe in optic canal
Probe in foramen rotundum
Sphenopalatine foramen
Lateral pterygoid plate
Probe in greater palatine canal
Frontal sinus
Orbital plate of frontal bone
Lacrimal bone
Fossa of lacrimal sac
Uncinate process of ethmoid bone
Maxillary process of inferior concha
Maxillary sinus
Alveolar process

©2014 Wolters Kluwer

Anatomy of the Teeth

30

Primary Teeth

Upper Teeth

A B C F G
6 7-8 16 12 24

Eruption, in months

Lower Teeth

24 12 16 G F C B A
6 7-8

Permanent Teeth

Upper Teeth

A B C D E F G H
7-8 13 10-12 6 12 18

Eruption, in years

Lower Teeth

H G F E D C B A
12 6 10-12 7-8

A Central incisor
B Lateral incisor
C Canine
D First premolar
E Second premolar
F First molar
G Second molar
H Third molar

Function of the Teeth

Incisor: Acts like scissors; grasps and cuts food.

Bicuspid: Has two pointed projections; tears, shreds, crushes food.

Cuspid: Has a single, very long, sharp cusp; tears and shreds food.

Molar: Strongest, most useful type of tooth; grinds food into tiny pieces.

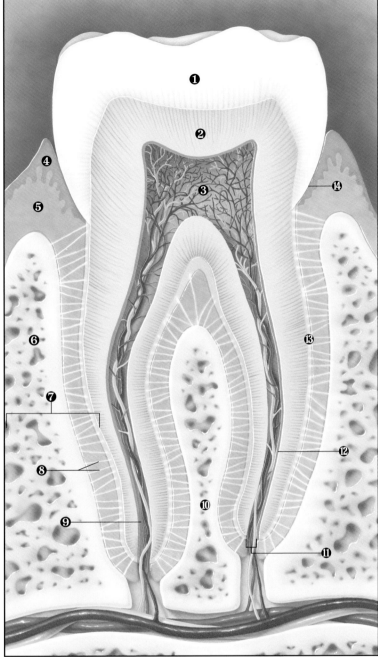

1 Enamel
2 Dentin, with dentinal tubules
3 Pulp chamber containing vessels and nerves
4 Gingival (gum) epithelium
5 Lamina propria of gingiva (gum)
6 Bone
7 Periodontium
8 Periodontal membranes
9 Root canal
10 Interradicular septum
11 Apical foramina
12 Odontoblast layer
13 Cementum
14 Gingival sulcus

Childhood Dentition

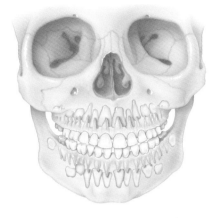

Beneath the erupted primary (baby or milk) teeth lie the permanent teeth (shown in blue). The twenty primary teeth are replaced as the child grows. Eruption and shedding dates are shown in the drawings on the far left.

Oral Cavity

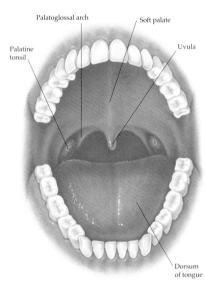

Palatoglossal arch
Soft palate
Palatine tonsil
Uvula
Dorsum of tongue

Tooth Decay

1 Decay of enamel
2 Decay invades dentin
3 Inflammation of pulp
4 Death of pulp
5 Abscess formation

Innervation and Blood Supply

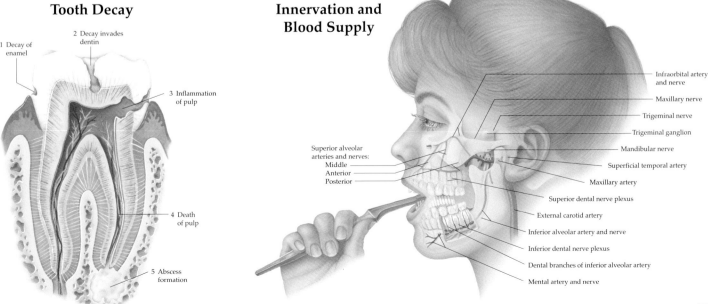

Infraorbital artery and nerve
Maxillary nerve
Trigeminal nerve
Trigeminal ganglion
Mandibular nerve
Superficial temporal artery
Maxillary artery
Superior dental nerve plexus
External carotid artery
Inferior alveolar artery and nerve
Inferior dental nerve plexus
Dental branches of inferior alveolar artery
Mental artery and nerve

Superior alveolar arteries and nerves:
Middle
Anterior
Posterior

©2014 Wolters Kluwer

The Vertebral Column

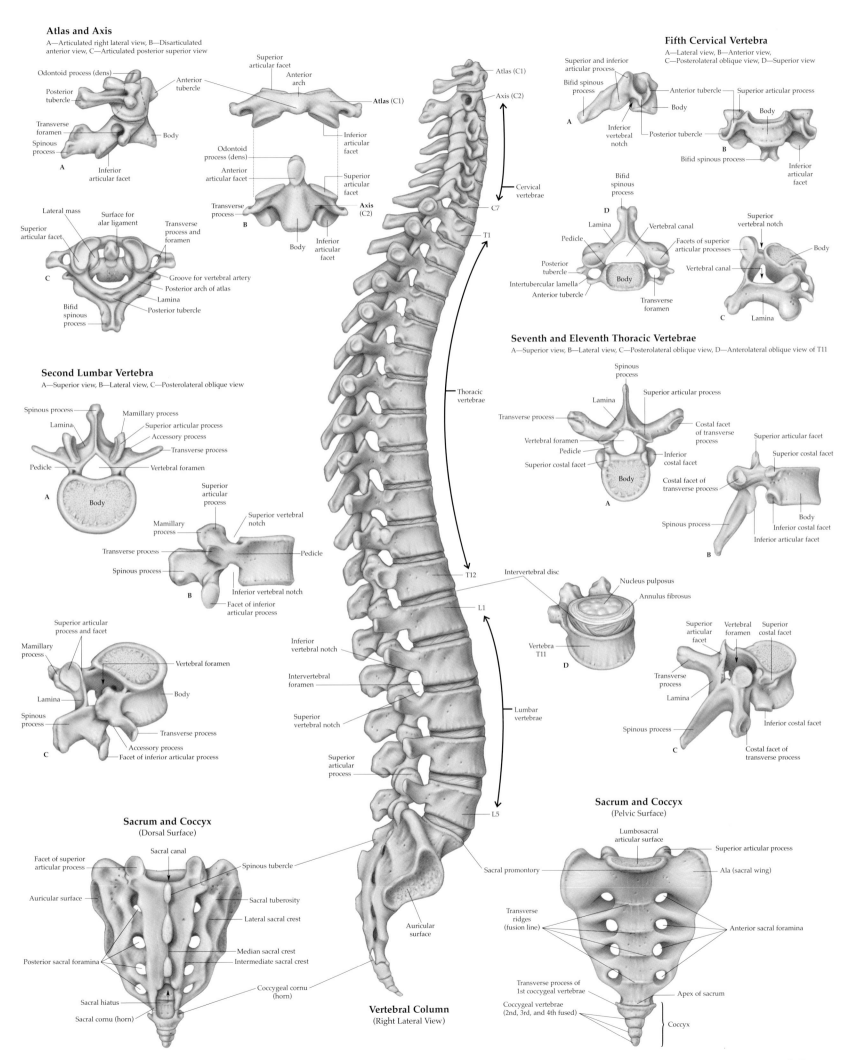

Atlas and Axis
A—Articulated right lateral view, B—Disarticulated anterior view, C—Articulated posterior superior view

Fifth Cervical Vertebra
A—Lateral view, B—Anterior view, C—Posterolateral oblique view, D—Superior view

Second Lumbar Vertebra
A—Superior view, B—Lateral view, C—Posterolateral oblique view

Seventh and Eleventh Thoracic Vertebrae
A—Superior view, B—Lateral view, C—Posterolateral oblique view, D—Anterolateral oblique view of T11

Sacrum and Coccyx
(Dorsal Surface)

Sacrum and Coccyx
(Pelvic Surface)

Vertebral Column
(Right Lateral View)

©2014 Wolters Kluwer

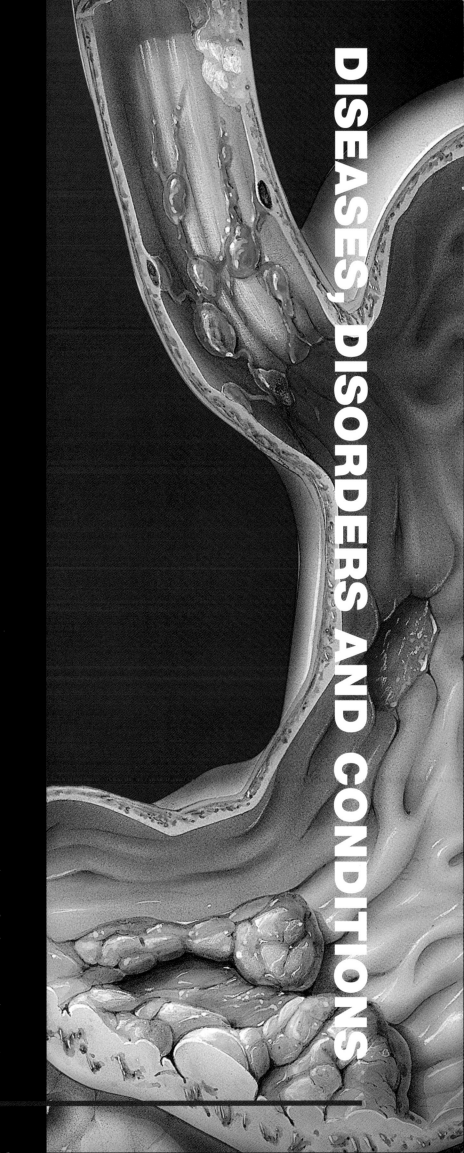

DISEASES, DISORDERS AND CONDITIONS

Dangers of Alcohol

The form of alcohol we drink is ethyl alcohol. It is made from sugar, starch, and other carbohydrates by the process of fermentation with yeast.

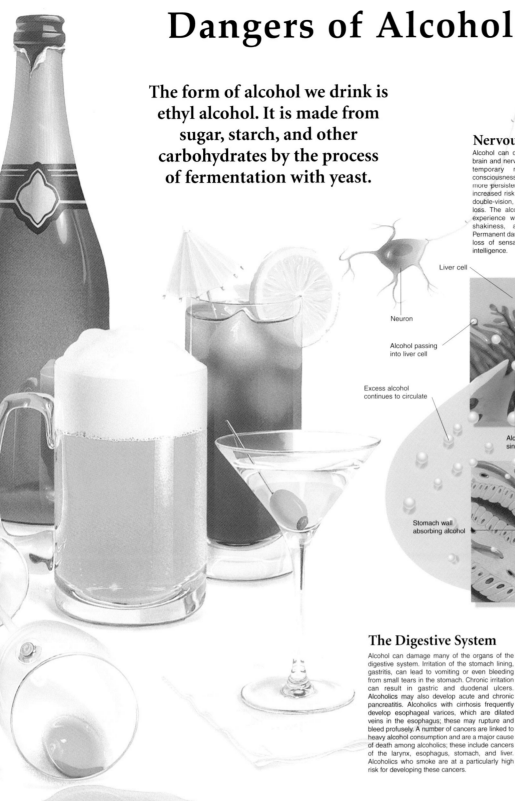

Nervous System

Alcohol can damage many body tissues including the brain and nerves. Excessive intake of alcohol can cause temporary memory loss (blackouts), loss of consciousness, or coma. Heavier drinkers may suffer with more persistent short-term memory loss and are at an increased risk of stroke. Chronic alcoholics may develop double-vision, loss of balance, and profound memory loss. The alcoholic who suddenly stops drinking may experience withdrawal symptoms, which can include shakiness, anxiety, hallucinations, and seizures. Permanent damage from alcoholism can include pain and loss of sensation in the arms and legs and loss of intelligence.

Neuron

Liver cell

Alcohol passing into liver cell

Excess alcohol continues to circulate

Hepatic sinusoid in liver tissue

Alcohol passing through sinusoid wall

Stomach wall absorbing alcohol

Alcohol Absorption

Alcohol is absorbed through the walls of the stomach and small intestine; it is carried by the blood vessels to the liver to be metabolized. Here, alcohol in the blood flows through the sinusoids, passes through the sinusoid walls, and enters the liver cells. The liver can only process about 1 oz of alcohol per hour, which is roughly equal to a standard drink; any excess amount will continue to circulate throughout the entire body until the liver is able to process more.

Esophageal cancer

Esophageal varices

Gastritis

Gastric ulcer

Duodenal ulcer

Stomach cancer

Pancreatitis

The Digestive System

Alcohol can damage many of the organs of the digestive system. Irritation of the stomach lining, gastritis, can lead to vomiting or even bleeding from small tears in the stomach. Chronic irritation can result in gastric and duodenal ulcers. Alcoholics may also develop acute and chronic pancreatitis. Alcoholics with cirrhosis frequently develop esophageal varices, which are dilated veins in the esophagus; these may rupture and bleed profusely. A number of cancers are linked to heavy alcohol consumption and are a major cause of death among alcoholics; these include cancers of the larynx, esophagus, stomach, and liver. Alcoholics who smoke are at a particularly high risk for developing these cancers.

Excessive drinking can lead to alcohol abuse and dependence, the disease of alcoholism. Some individuals may be genetically predisposed to alcoholism. Consequences of the misuse of alcohol include destroyed relationships, loss of job, poor health, and death.

However, moderate alcohol consumption may have health benefits, particularly in preventing cardiovascular disease. Moderate drinking is defined as two drinks (or less) a day for males under 65 years of age and one drink (or less) per day for males over the age of 65 years and females.

Complications

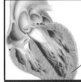

Damaged and weakened heart muscle

Heart Disease

Short-term effects from a drink may include an increased pulse rate and dilation of blood vessels. Chronic alcohol use can cause serious damage such as high blood pressure and cardiomyopathy, a damaged and weakened heart muscle. Heavy drinkers are also at risk for an abnormal heart rhythm.

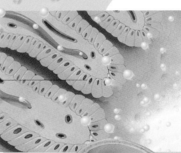

Cirrhosis

Lipid droplets increased

Liver cell in fatty liver disease

Normal liver cell

Liver Disease

The liver is frequently affected in chronic alcohol abuse. Consequences may include fatty liver disease (an accumulation of fat droplets inside liver cells), alcohol induced hepatitis, and cirrhosis. In cirrhosis, liver cells die and scar tissue irreversibly changes the normal architecture of the liver tissue.

Alcohol passing through placental barrier

Maternal blood

Fetal blood vessels

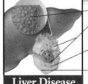

Reproduction

Excessive alcohol consumption may cause impotence and damage to sperm in men. For women, alcohol use may cause interruptions in menstruation and damage to eggs. Alcohol may also cause serious problems for the developing fetus that can affect its entire life. The baby can be born with fetal alcohol syndrome, be underweight, grow slower, and have birth defects, as well as have a smaller brain and a lower IQ, or mental retardation. Alcohol may be passed to a baby through breast milk as well.

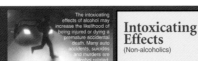

Intoxication: The blood alcohol concentration (the amount of alcohol in the blood) roughly correlates with the level of mental and physical impairment (intoxication). The level of alcohol measured in breath tests closely parallels the blood alcohol concentration. Given the same amount of alcohol, levels from person to person can vary depending on body weight, body fat, recent meals, tolerance, and how quickly the alcohol was consumed. Women and older individuals tend to be more sensitive to the effects of alcohol. Once alcohol is in your blood, the only effective cure for intoxication is time. The legal limit for driving in all U.S. states is 80 mg/dL or 0.08 percent.

The intoxicating effects of alcohol may increase the likelihood of being injured or dying a premature accidental death. Many auto accidents, suicides, and murders are alcohol related.

Intoxicating Effects
(Non-alcoholics)

More than 25 mg/dL or 0.025 percent (blood alcohol concentration)	More than 100mg/dL or 0.1 percent (blood alcohol concentration)	If alcohol levels continue to rise...
• Mild intoxication • Altered mood • Impaired thinking • Incoordination	• Decreased inhibition • Euphoria followed by depression • Hostility • Slurred speech • Double vision	• Stupor • Coma

©2014 Wolters Kluwer

Understanding Allergies

What Is An Allergy?

An allergy is an overreaction or hypersensitivity of the body's immune system to normally harmless substances, called allergens. An allergic reaction occurs when the body's immune system responds to an allergen as if the substance were disease causing. Subsequent exposures to this substance can result in physical symptoms that range from mild to life threatening.

Who Gets Allergies?

The tendency to develop allergies is thought to be inherited, because they commonly develop in those who have a family history of allergies. It is possible for anyone to develop allergies at any age. Environmental factors can make our immune systems overly sensitive. This could then trigger allergies in people with no family history or hasten the onset in those with a family history.

What Are Common Allergens?

Allergens can enter the body in a number of different ways, including inhaling, eating/drinking, injection (as with bee venom), and contact with the skin or eyes. Common allergens include pollen, mold, animal hair or dander, dust mites, certain medications (for example, penicillin), and certain foods (for example, peanuts, eggs, milk, wheat, and seafood).

Anaphylaxis: An Allergic Emergency

Anaphylaxis is a life-threatening reaction. The onset of this reaction may occur within seconds or minutes of exposure. Symptoms may include a red rash over most of the body. Skin becomes warm to the touch, intense tightening and swelling of the airways make breathing difficult, and there is a drop in blood pressure. Breathing can stop and the body may slip into shock. If medication is not administered quickly, heart failure and death can result within minutes in the most severe reactions. Allergens in insect venom and medications such as antibiotics are more likely to cause anaphylaxis than are any other allergens. Anaphylaxis is not a common reaction and can be controlled with prompt medication and the help of a physician.

Managing Allergies

The first step in managing allergies is to identify the type of reaction you are having, whether it is watery eyes, sneezing, or difficulty breathing. Second, try to identify the trigger or the situation that led to the symptoms. Ask yourself a few questions:

- *Where did the reaction occur?*
- *Inside or outside?*
- *Were you eating or drinking?*
- *Were there any animals or insects near you?*
- *Were you wearing any new clothing?*
- *Did you use a new soap or detergent?*

A physician can perform skin or blood allergy tests with a variety of common allergens. Once the allergen has been identified, manage your allergies by following some tips:

- *Avoid allergens when possible.*
- *Avoid tobacco smoke and other irritants.*
- *Use medication as prescribed.*
- *See a doctor regularly.*
- *Stay healthy.*

Seafood

Drugs

Peanuts

Mold

Pollen

Dander   Dust mites

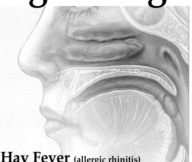

Hay Fever (allergic rhinitis)

Commonly caused by exposure to ragweed and some tree pollens. It affects the eyes and nose. Causes sneezing; runny nose; watery, itchy eyes; irritated, itchy throat; and sometimes, a stuffy, blocked nose.

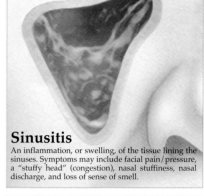

Sinusitis

An inflammation, or swelling, of the tissue lining the sinuses. Symptoms may include facial pain/pressure, a "stuffy head" (congestion), nasal stuffiness, nasal discharge, and loss of sense of smell.

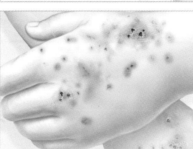

Eczema (atopic dermatitis)

A group of medical conditions that cause the skin to become inflamed or irritated. It causes itchy, red rashes of the skin characterized by lesions, scaling, and flaking.

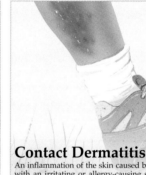

Hives (urticaria)

An outbreak of swollen, pale red bumps or patches (wheals) on the skin, as a result of the body's adverse reaction to certain allergens, or for unknown reasons.

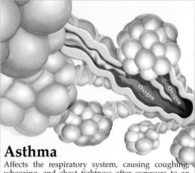

Asthma

Affects the respiratory system, causing coughing, wheezing, and chest tightness after exposure to an allergen. Common allergens that worsen asthma include plant pollens and dust mites.

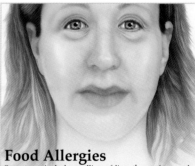

Contact Dermatitis

An inflammation of the skin caused by direct contact with an irritating or allergy-causing substance (such as poison ivy or latex gloves). It causes redness, itching, swelling, or rashes on the skin.

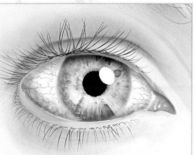

Allergic Conjunctivitis

An inflammation of the conjunctiva, the tissue that lines the eyeball and inside of the eyelid, associated with allergies. The eye becomes red, itchy, and watery.

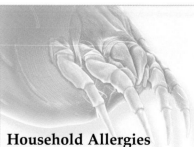

Food Allergies

Symptoms include swelling of lips, throat, face, and tongue; upset stomach; vomiting; abdominal cramps; hives; and skin rashes. Food allergies may be life threatening.

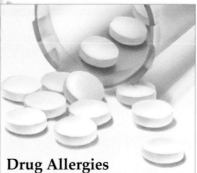

Drug Allergies

Certain medicines can trigger allergic reactions ranging from mild rashes to life-threatening symptoms, which can affect any tissue or organ in the body.

Household Allergies

Dust mites are microscopic organisms that feed on live and shed skin tissue. Mites are commonly found on pillows, mattresses, and upholstered furniture. Mite feces are responsible for a majority of the year-round types of allergies, and are a major cause of asthma.

©2014 Wolters Kluwer

Osteoarthritis (OA)

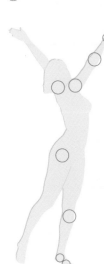

- Most common type of arthritis.
- Primarily affects cartilage, the tissue that cushions the ends of bones within the joints.
- May initially affect joints asymmetrically.
- Affects hands and weight bearing joints.
- Can cause joint pain and stiffness.
- Usually develops slowly over many years.

◯ = identifies areas most affected by OA.

Rheumatoid Arthritis (RA)

- Causes redness, warmth, and swelling of joints.
- Usually affects the same joint on both sides of the body.
- Often causes a general feeling of sickness, fatigue, weight loss, and fever.
- May develop suddenly, within weeks or months.
- Most often begins between ages 25 and 50.

◯ = identifies areas most affected by RA.

Other Arthritic Diseases

Many people use the word *arthritis* to refer to all rheumatic diseases. However, the word literally means joint inflammation. Other types of arthritis include:

Fibromyalgia (Fibrositis)

- Chronic disorder that causes pain throughout the tissues that support and move the bones and joints.
- Pain, stiffness, and localized tender points occur in the muscles and tendons, particularly those of the spine, shoulders, and hips.
- Patients may also experience fatigue and sleep disturbances.

Gout

- Results from deposits of needle-like crystals of uric acid in the joints.
- The crystals cause inflammation, swelling, and pain in the affected joint, which is often the big toe.

Juvenile Rheumatoid Arthritis

- Most common form of arthritis in children.
- Causes pain, stiffness, swelling, and impaired function of the joints.
- May be associated with rashes or fevers; may affect various parts of the body.

Systemic Lupus Erythematosus

- Also known as *lupus* or *SLE*.
- Can result in inflammation of and damage to the joints, skin, kidneys, heart, lungs, blood vessels, and brain.

Bursitis

- Inflammation of a bursa, a small, fluid-filled sac that absorbs shock and reduces friction around a joint.
- May be caused by arthritis in the joint or by injury or infection of the bursa.
- Produces pain and tenderness and may limit the movement of nearby joints.

Tendinitis

- Inflammation of a tendon, a cord of fibrous tissue that attaches muscle to bone.
- May be caused by overuse, injury, or a rheumatic condition.
- Produces pain and tenderness and may restrict movement of nearby joints.

Common Symptoms of Arthritis

- Swelling in one or more joints.
- Stiffness around the joints (each episode of stiffness for RA lasts one hour or more, but OA lasts 30 minutes or less).
- Constant or recurring pain or tenderness in a joint.
- Difficulty using or moving a joint normally.
- Warmth and redness in a joint.

If you have any of these symptoms for more than two weeks, contact your physician.

Joints Affected by Osteoarthritis (OA)

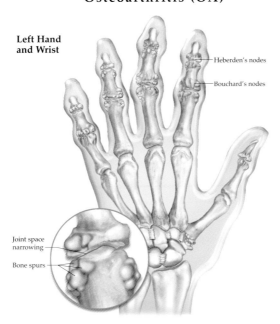

Left Hand and Wrist

Heberden's nodes
Bouchard's nodes

Joint space narrowing
Bone spurs

Joints Affected by Rheumatoid Arthritis (RA)

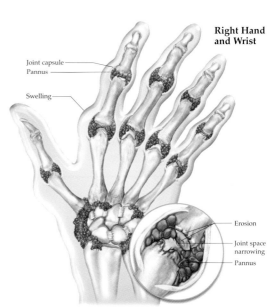

Right Hand and Wrist

Joint capsule
Pannus
Swelling
Erosion
Joint space narrowing
Pannus

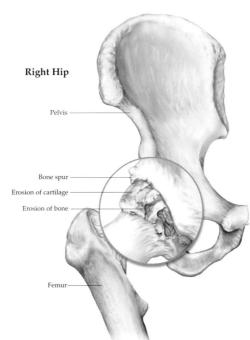

Right Hip

Pelvis
Bone spur
Erosion of cartilage
Erosion of bone
Femur

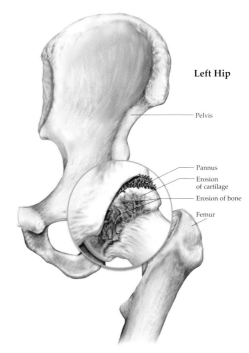

Left Hip

Pelvis
Pannus
Erosion of cartilage
Erosion of bone
Femur

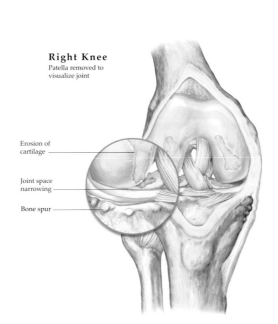

Right Knee
Patella removed to visualize joint

Erosion of cartilage
Joint space narrowing
Bone spur

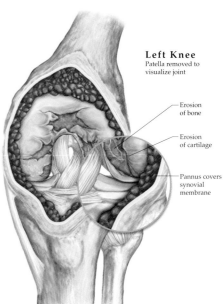

Left Knee
Patella removed to visualize joint

Erosion of bone
Erosion of cartilage
Pannus covers synovial membrane

©2014 Wolters Kluwer

Understanding Asthma

What Happens in an Asthma Attack?

What Is Asthma?

Asthma is a chronic disease of the lungs in which inflammation causes the airways to narrow, making breathing more difficult.

What Causes Asthma?

Although the actual cause of asthma is not known, many studies have shown that it may be due to a combination of factors. We do know that asthma is not contagious like the flu. We also know that people have a higher risk of developing asthma if a family member has had an asthma attack or if they live with people who smoke.

How Is Asthma Diagnosed?

There is no single or definitive test for asthma. It is diagnosed based on a review of the patient's medical history and those of his or her family. There are many tests your doctor may use to get more information about your condition. These include pulmonary function tests, allergy tests, blood tests, and chest and sinus x-rays.

A Smooth muscle tightens the airways.

Smooth muscle

Alveoli

B Sides of airways have become inflamed and swollen, making it harder for oxygen to get to alveoli.

C Excess mucus has formed inside the airways.

Sides of airways are thin to allow more space for oxygen to get to alveoli.

Bronchiole During an Asthma Attack

Healthy Bronchiole

How Do the Lungs Work?

When you breathe, you draw in (inhale) fresh air and oxygen into your lungs and expel (exhale) stale air and carbon dioxide from your lungs.

1 The incoming air goes through a network of airways (bronchial tubes) that reach the lungs.

2 As the air moves through the lungs, the bronchial tubes become progressively smaller, like branches of a tree.

3 At the end of the smallest tubes are alveolar sacs, the site of gas exchange between the lungs and the circulatory system.

4 Oxygen enters the alveolar sacs, where it passes to the bloodstream and is then used by the body.

5 Carbon dioxide (waste product) from the bloodstream enters the alveolar sacs to be carried out of the lungs.

Monitoring Your Asthma by Zone

Green Zone	Yellow Zone	Red Zone
No asthma symptoms. Able to do usual activities and sleep without coughing, wheezing, or breathing difficulty.	There may be coughing, wheezing, and mild shortness of breath. Sleep and usual activities may be disturbed. May be more tired than usual.	Symptoms may include frequent, severe cough; severe shortness of breath; wheezing; trouble talking while walking; rapid breathing.
Action: Keep controlling/preventing your asthma symptoms. Continue to take your asthma medicines exactly as prescribed by your healthcare specialist, even if you have no symptoms and feel fine.	**Action:** Keep controlling your asthma symptoms and add your prescribed quick-relief medicine. Call to discuss the situation with your doctor or healthcare specialist.	**Action:** Go to an emergency room.

Symptoms of Asthma

Symptoms of asthma often vary from time to time in an individual. The severity of an asthma attack can increase rapidly, so it is important to treat your symptoms immediately once you recognize them.

Adult Symptoms
• Wheezing
• Chest tightness
• Coughing
• Difficulty breathing: shortness of breath

Childhood Symptoms
• Coughing at night or during sleep
• Diminished responsiveness
• Constant rattly cough
• Frequent chest colds
• Rapid breathing
• Weak cry
• Grunt when nursing or have difficulty feeding
• Chest might feel "funny"
• Unexplained irritability

Common Asthma Triggers

The airways in an asthmatic person are extremely sensitive to certain factors known as triggers. When stimulated by these triggers, the airways overreact with abnormal inflammation that leads to swelling, increased mucus secretion, and muscle contraction of the air passages. Examples of asthma triggers include:

• Pollution: cigarette smoke,* smog, strong odors from painting or cooking, scented products
• Allergens: animal dander, dust mites, cockroaches, pollen, mold
• Cold air or changes in weather
• Illness and infections
• Exercise
• Medications such as pain relievers
• Sulfites or other additives in food and beverages
• GERD (gastroesophageal reflux disease)

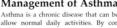

The proteins on dust mites are among the allergens that may trigger an asthma attack.

People can have trouble with one or more triggers. Your doctor can help you identify your asthma triggers and ways to avoid them.

*The risk of asthma is increased in children who are regularly exposed to cigarette smoke.

Management of Asthma

Asthma is a chronic disease that can be controlled to allow normal daily activities. By controlling your asthma every day, you can prevent serious symptoms and take part in all activities. If your asthma is not well controlled, you are likely to have symptoms that can make you miss school or work and keep you from doing other things you enjoy. Although there is no cure, here are some important prevention strategies:

• Recognize attacks early.
• Take medication as directed.
• Avoid tobacco smoke.
• Identify and avoid triggers.
• Talk with your doctor to find ways to improve your health.
• Get the influenza vaccination (flu shot) every year and a pneumococcal vaccination (pneumonia shot) every five years.

©2014 Wolters Kluwer

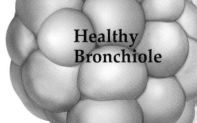

Understanding High Blood Pressure

Complications of High Blood Pressure

High Blood pressure that is not controlled can cause long-term damage to your blood vessels, brain, heart, kidneys, and eyes. Learning about your blood pressure can help reduce your risk of having a stroke or heart attack. Ask your health care provider to check your blood pressure today.

BRAIN

Stroke – Blood vessels in the brain that are damaged, weakened and narrowed by high blood pressure may bulge out (aneurysm) and burst causing blood to seep into the brain tissue (hemorrhage). Or blood clots may form in the arteries leading to the brain, blocking blood flow.
Transient Ischemic Attack – TIA (mini stroke) is a brief, temporary disruption of blood supply to the brain. It's often caused by atherosclerosis or a blood clot — both of which can be a result of high blood pressure.

Hemorrhage   Blood clot   Aneurysm at junction of main arteries of the brain

EYES

Thickened, narrowed or torn blood vessels in the eyes may result in vision loss.

Damaged blood vessels in the retina of the eye

BLOOD VESSELS

High blood pressure can damage the inner walls of arteries causing them to thicken and harden, a condition called **arteriosclerosis**. Cholesterol and other substances (plaque) in the blood can collect on the damaged walls of the arteries; a condition called **atherosclerosis**; and may block blood flow causing problems such as chest pain (angina), heart attack, heart failure, kidney failure, stroke, blocked arteries in your legs or arms (peripheral arterial disease), eye damage, and aneurysms.

Thickened artery walls   Plaque buildup on walls of artery
Arteriosclerosis   Atherosclerosis

ANEURYSM

Over time, the constant pressure of blood moving through a weakened artery can cause a section of its wall to enlarge and form a bulge (aneurysm). An aneurysm can burst and cause internal bleeding. Aneurysms can form in any artery in the body, but they're most common in the aorta, the body's largest artery.

Aortic aneurysm   Burst aneurysm

HEART

Coronary Artery Disease (CAD) – Affects the arteries that supply blood to the heart. Thickened and narrowed coronary arteries prevent blood from flowing freely to the heart, causing chest pain (angina), heart attack or irregular heart rhythms (arrhythmias).
Left Ventricular Hypertrophy (LVH) – High blood pressure forces the heart to work harder to pump blood to the rest of the body. This causes the heart's left pumping chamber (the left ventricle) to thicken or stiffen limiting the ventricle's ability to pump blood, increasing the risk of heart attack, heart failure and sudden cardiac death.
Heart failure – Over time, the strain on the heart from high blood pressure can cause the heart to weaken and work less efficiently, eventually failing to meet the body's demand for blood.

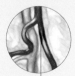

Blocked coronary arteries   Thickened heart muscle
Angina   Left Ventricular Hypertrophy

KIDNEYS

High blood pressure is one of the most common causes of kidney failure. It can damage both the large arteries leading to the kidneys and the tiny blood vessels within the kidneys. Damage to either prevents the kidneys from effectively filtering waste from the blood, allowing dangerous levels of fluid and waste to accumulate.

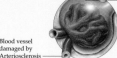

Glomerulus – filters waste from blood

Blood vessel damaged by Arteriosclerosis

Prevention and Management

High blood pressure can be prevented and managed best by adjusting your lifestyle. Decrease your blood pressure by:

- Reduce body weight if overweight
- Maintain a healthy weight
- Eat healthy foods
- Decrease salt in your diet
- Decrease fat in your diet
- Increase fiber in your diet
- Do not smoke
- Avoid excessive alcohol intake
- Exercise regularly
- Manage stress
- Follow your physician's instructions and take any medications as prescribed

What is High Blood Pressure?

When the heart beats, it pumps blood out to all parts of the body thru the arteries creating force or pressure against the walls of the arteries. Like air in a tire, blood fills arteries to a certain capacity. But just as too much air pressure can damage a tire, high blood pressure can damage healthy arteries. When blood pressure is high the heart must work harder to pump the same amount of blood through the arteries. Blood pressure rises and falls during the day, but when blood pressure stays high over time, it is called high blood pressure (HBP) or hypertension. The wear and tear caused by untreated high blood pressure can cause damage to the heart, kidneys and eyes, and increases the risk for heart attack, stroke, kidney failure, coronary artery disease, and other serious health problems.

Signs and Symptoms of High Blood Pressure

Most of the time, high blood pressure does not cause any symptoms. It is often diagnosed when a patient visits their physician for a routine check-up. Many people do not realize they have high blood pressure until it has caused damage to their body. In rare cases, headaches can result from extremely high blood pressure.

How is Blood Pressure Measured?

Blood pressure is measured with a simple test using a blood pressure cuff. The cuff is wrapped around your upper arm and inflated enough to stop the blood flow in your artery for a few seconds. When the cuff is released or deflated, the first sound heard by your health care provider through the stethoscope is the whooshing sound of your heart pushing blood into your arteries. This is called the "systolic" blood pressure. The "diastolic" blood pressure is when this noise disappears, indicating the heart is relaxed. The systolic blood pressure number is always stated first followed by the diastolic number. For example, your blood pressure may be read as "117 over 76", or written "117/76".

Two numbers are used to describe blood pressure:

117 / 76 mm Hg

Systolic (top number) The top number called "systolic blood pressure" measures blood pressure when the heart pumps blood forward through the arteries to the rest of your body. This force creates pressure on the arteries. Blood pressure is highest when the heart beats, pumping the blood. A normal healthy number is around 117.

mmHg is a measurement of pressure

Diastolic (bottom number) The second number is lower than the systolic pressure and measures blood pressure when the heart relaxes between beats. This is called "diastolic blood pressure." A normal healthy number is around 76. Your blood pressure normally changes throughout the day. It rises when you are active, and lowers when you are resting.

Healthy and Unhealthy Blood Pressure Levels

Blood Pressure Category	Systolic mm Hg (upper #)		Diastolic mm Hg (lower #)
Normal	less than **120**	and	less than **80**
Prehypertension	**120 – 139**	or	**80 – 89**
High Blood Pressure (Hypertension) **Stage 1**	**140 – 159**	or	**90 – 99**
High Blood Pressure (Hypertension) **Stage 2**	**160** or higher	or	**100** or higher
Hypertensive Crisis (Emergency care needed)	Higher than **180**	or	Higher than **110**

http://www.heart.org/HEARTORG/   *Your doctor should evaluate unusually low blood pressure readings.*

Types and Causes of High Blood Pressure (Hypertension)

Primary or essential hypertension is the most common type of high blood pressure. In most cases the exact causes are unknown; however there are several factors that increase or contribute to your chances of developing high blood pressure:

- Obesity or being overweight
- Lack of physical activity
- Poor diet, especially one that includes too much salt and too little potassium
- Genetics and family medical history
- Age and gender
- High levels of alcohol consumption
- Ethnic background
- Stress
- Smoking and second hand smoke

Secondary hypertension may result from a known cause such as:

- Chronic kidney disease
- Adrenal and thyroid problems or tumors
- Diabetes
- Pregnancy
- Some neurologic disorders

High Blood Pressure in Children

Teens, children and even babies can have high blood pressure. Although high blood pressure is far more common among adults, the rate among kids is on the rise, a trend that experts link to the increase in childhood obesity. Early diagnosis and treatment can reduce or prevent the harmful complications of high blood pressure. The American Heart Association recommends that all children have their blood pressure measured yearly. Children have the same test for high blood pressure as adults; however, interpreting the numbers is more difficult. Your child's physician will use charts based on your child's gender, height, age and blood pressure numbers to determine whether or not your child has high blood pressure.

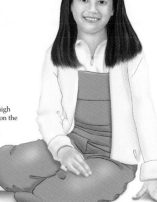

©2014 Wolters Kluwer

Understanding Breast Cancer

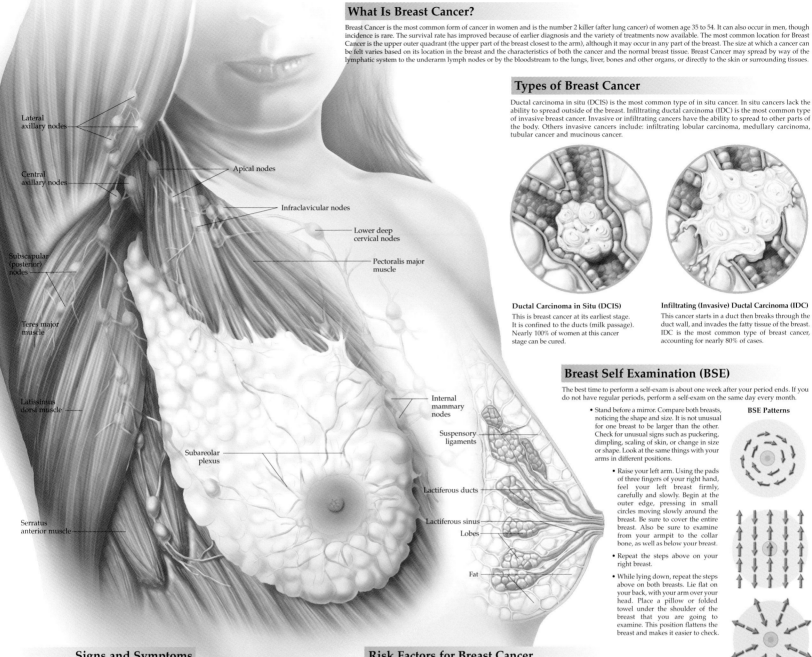

What Is Breast Cancer?

Breast Cancer is the most common form of cancer in women and is the number 2 killer (after lung cancer) of women age 35 to 54. It can also occur in men, though incidence is rare. The survival rate has improved because of earlier diagnosis and the variety of treatments now available. The most common location for Breast Cancer is the upper outer quadrant (the upper part of the breast closest to the arm), although it may occur in any part of the breast. The size at which a cancer can be felt varies based on its location in the breast and the characteristics of both the cancer and the normal breast tissue. Breast Cancer may spread by way of the lymphatic system to the underarm lymph nodes or by the bloodstream to the lungs, liver, bones and other organs, or directly to the skin or surrounding tissues.

Types of Breast Cancer

Ductal carcinoma in situ (DCIS) is the most common type of in situ cancer. In situ cancers lack the ability to spread outside of the breast. Infiltrating ductal carcinoma (IDC) is the most common type of invasive breast cancer. Invasive or infiltrating cancers have the ability to spread to other parts of the body. Others invasive cancers include: infiltrating lobular carcinoma, medullary carcinoma, tubular cancer and mucinous cancer.

Ductal Carcinoma in Situ (DCIS)
This is breast cancer at its earliest stage. It is confined to the ducts (milk passage). Nearly 100% of women at this cancer stage can be cured.

Infiltrating (Invasive) Ductal Carcinoma (IDC)
This cancer starts in a duct then breaks through the duct wall, and invades the fatty tissue of the breast. IDC is the most common type of breast cancer, accounting for nearly 80% of cases.

Breast Self Examination (BSE)

The best time to perform a self-exam is about one week after your period ends. If you do not have regular periods, perform a self-exam on the same day every month.

- Stand before a mirror. Compare both breasts, noticing the shape and size. It is not unusual for one breast to be larger than the other. Check for unusual signs such as puckering, dimpling, scaling of skin, or change in size or shape. Look at the same things with your arms in different positions.

- Raise your left arm. Using the pads of three fingers of your right hand, feel your left breast firmly, carefully and slowly. Begin at the outer edge, pressing in small circles moving slowly around the breast. Be sure to cover the entire breast. Also be sure to examine from your armpit to the collar bone, as well as below your breast.

- Repeat the steps above on your right breast.

- While lying down, repeat the steps above on both breasts. Lie flat on your back, with your arm over your head. Place a pillow or folded towel under the shoulder of the breast that you are going to examine. This position flattens the breast and makes it easier to check.

BSE Patterns

Signs and Symptoms

- A lump or mass in the breast
- Change in shape or size of the breast
- Change in the skin, such as thickening or dimpling, scaly skin around the nipple, an orange-peel-like appearance, or ulcers
- Discharge from the nipple that occurs without squeezing the nipple
- Change in the nipple, such as itching, burning, erosion, or retraction
- Swelling of the arm
- Pain (with an advanced tumor)
- Change in skin temperature or color (a warm, hot, or pink area)

Risk Factors for Breast Cancer

The cause of breast cancer isn't known, but its higher incidence in women suggests that estrogen is a cause or contributing factor. Women who are at increased risk include those who:

- have a family history of breast cancer in close relatives (mother, sister, daughter)
- have a long menstrual history (began menstruating at an early age or experienced menopause late)
- have had cancer in one breast
- have had breast biopsy showing atypical hyperplasia (increased cell production)
- were first pregnant after age 31
- have never been pregnant
- were exposed to low-level ionizing radiation

Staging

Clinical Staging is a part of the pretreatment evaluation and is performed based on physical exam and x-rays studies. The final (pathologic) stage is determined by microscopic examination of the biopsied tissue and axillary specimen to assess the size of the cancer and the presence of lymph node involvement, and the possibility of systemic metastasis (spread of cancer outside of the breast and lymph nodes). The most commonly used system is the **Tumor-Nodes-Metastasis system (TNM)**. **T** represents the tumor, **N** the lymph node involvement, and **M** the metastasis if any.

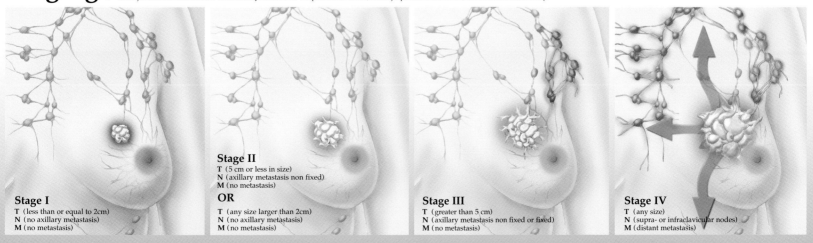

Stage I
T (less than or equal to 2cm)
N (no axillary metastasis)
M (no metastasis)

Stage II
T (5 cm or less in size)
N (axillary metastasis non fixed)
M (no metastasis)
OR
T (any size larger than 2cm)
N (no axillary metastasis)
M (no metastasis)

Stage III
T (greater than 5 cm)
N (axillary metastasis non fixed or fixed)
M (no metastasis)

Stage IV
T (any size)
N (supra- or infraclavicular nodes)
M (distant metastasis)

©2014 Wolters Kluwer

Cardiovascular Disease

NORMAL HEART ANATOMY

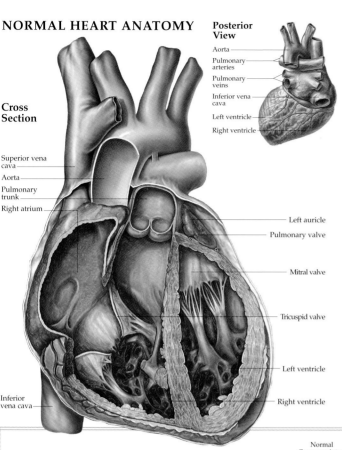

Cross Section

- Superior vena cava
- Aorta
- Pulmonary trunk
- Right atrium
- Left auricle
- Pulmonary valve
- Mitral valve
- Tricuspid valve
- Left ventricle
- Inferior vena cava
- Right ventricle

Posterior View

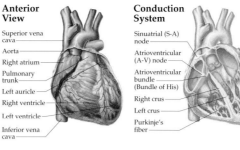

- Aorta
- Pulmonary arteries
- Pulmonary veins
- Inferior vena cava
- Left ventricle
- Right ventricle

Anterior View

- Superior vena cava
- Aorta
- Right atrium
- Pulmonary trunk
- Left auricle
- Right ventricle
- Left ventricle
- Inferior vena cava

Conduction System

- Sinuatrial (S-A) node
- Atrioventricular (A-V) node
- Atrioventricular bundle (Bundle of His)
- Right crus
- Left crus
- Purkinje's fiber

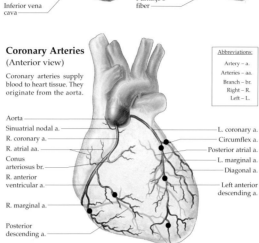

Coronary Arteries (Anterior view)

Coronary arteries supply blood to heart tissue. They originate from the aorta.

Abbreviations:
- Artery – a.
- Arteries – aa.
- Branch – br.
- Right – R.
- Left – L.

- Aorta
- Sinuatrial nodal a.
- R. coronary a.
- R. atrial aa.
- Conus arteriosus br.
- R. anterior ventricular a.
- R. marginal a.
- Posterior descending a.
- L. coronary a.
- Circumflex a.
- Posterior atrial a.
- L. marginal a.
- Diagonal a.
- Left anterior descending a.

● *Common areas of coronary artery blockage that result in damage to heart muscle.*

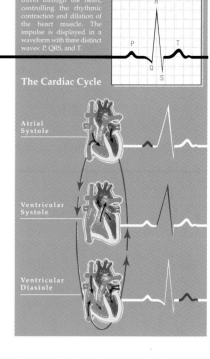

Electrocardiogram (ECG)

Repeating electrical impulses travel through the heart, controlling the rhythmic contraction and dilation of the heart muscle. The impulse is displayed in a waveform with three distinct waves: P, QRS, and T.

The Cardiac Cycle

- Atrial Systole
- Ventricular Systole
- Ventricular Diastole

CARDIOVASCULAR DISEASE

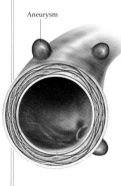

Aneurysm

Polyarteritis Nodosa (PAN)

Polyarteritis nodosa (PAN) is a disease of inflammation of the small and medium-sized blood vessels, which can involve multiple organs of the body. The organs most commonly involved are the kidneys, heart, liver, and gastrointestinal tract. Less commonly involved are the muscles, brain, spinal cord, peripheral nerves, and skin. The inflammation can cause beadlike aneurysms of the involved blood vessels, which cause decreased blood flow to the affected organs.

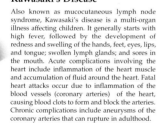

Inflammation of blood vessel

Kawasaki's Disease

Also known as mucocutaneous lymph node syndrome, Kawasaki's disease is a multi-organ illness affecting children. It generally starts with high fever, followed by the development of redness and swelling of the hands, feet, eyes, lips, and tongue; swollen lymph glands; and sores in the mouth. Acute complications involving the heart include inflammation of the heart muscle and accumulation of fluid around the heart. Fatal heart attacks occur due to inflammation of the blood vessels (coronary arteries) of the heart, causing blood clots to form and block the arteries. Chronic complications include aneurysms of the coronary arteries that can rupture in adulthood.

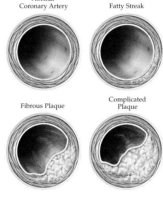

Normal Coronary Artery — Fatty Streak

Fibrous Plaque — Complicated Plaque

Coronary Artery Disease

If excessive amounts of fat are circulating in the blood, the arteries can accumulate fatty deposits called plaques. This buildup, called atherosclerosis, causes the vessels to narrow or become obstructed. Coronary artery disease results as atherosclerotic plaque fills the lumens of the coronary arteries and obstructs blood flow to the heart. This results in diminished supply of oxygen and nutrients to the heart tissue.

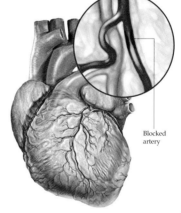

Blocked artery

Angina

The coronary arteries supplying the heart can become narrowed over time, due to age, hereditary factors, chronic smoking, high cholesterol, high blood pressure, or diabetes. The narrowed blood vessels limit the amount of blood flow to the heart, especially with strenuous activity. When the heart muscle is not getting enough blood, pain or discomfort in the chest, commonly called angina, results.

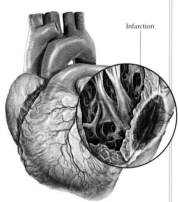

Infarction

Myocardial Infarction (Heart Attack)

Myocardial infarction occurs when a coronary artery narrowed by atherosclerosis becomes completely blocked. This is usually the result of a blood clot that forms where the artery is narrowed. The blocked artery prevents the heart from receiving oxygen, and part or all of the heart muscle is either damaged (infarction) or dies. The damaged part of the heart loses its ability to contract and pump blood to and from the heart.

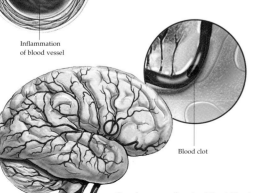

Blood clot

Cerebrovascular Accident (Stroke)

A cerebrovascular accident (CVA), also known as a stroke, is a sudden impairment of cerebral circulation in one or more blood vessels. This interrupts or diminishes oxygen supply to the brain, often causing the brain tissues to become damaged or die.

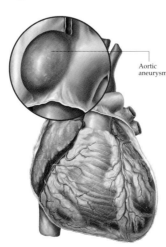

Aortic aneurysm

Aortic Aneurysm

The aorta is the largest blood vessel in the body. It comes out of the top of the heart and brings blood to the rest of the body. Atherosclerosis can cause the wall of the aorta to weaken and balloon out (aneurysm). The aortic aneurysm may suddenly rupture or tear, often leading to death.

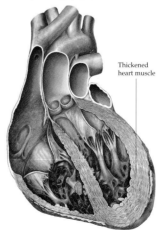

Thickened heart muscle

Left Ventricular Hypertrophy (LVH)

LVH is when the muscle of the heart's left ventricle becomes thickened and enlarged. The heart then becomes less efficient at circulating blood throughout the body. The resulting condition is called congestive heart failure. This may cause the lungs to fill up with fluid, resulting in difficulty breathing, fluid retention and swollen legs, and decreased blood flow to various parts of the body.

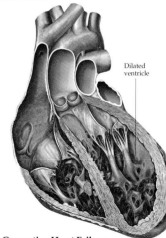

Dilated ventricle

Congestive Heart Failure

Congestive heart failure is a common debilitating condition defined by the heart's mechanical inability to pump blood effectively. The result is a decrease in blood circulation, which forces blood to back up and oxygen supply to decrease in muscle and lung tissues. Excess accumulation of fluids in tissues throughout the body causes swelling (edema), which impairs the function of affected organs.

©2014 Wolters Kluwer

Understanding High Cholesterol

What is High Cholesterol?

Cholesterol is a waxy, fat-like substance found in all of your body's cells. Cholesterol comes from two sources, your body and your food. Cholesterol is made in the liver and other cells and is also found in food from animals, like dairy products, eggs, and meat. You can end up with high cholesterol because of the foods you eat and the rate at which your body breaks down cholesterol. Your body needs a certain amount of cholesterol to build and maintain cells, but too much or too little cholesterol can create a major health risk. Extra cholesterol can build up on your artery walls and over time, cholesterol deposits, called plaque, may narrow your arteries causing less blood flow or form a clot, putting you at risk for heart disease, heart attack and stroke.

What Causes High Cholesterol?

- **Eating an unhealthy diet**
  – with too much saturated fat, trans fat, and cholesterol. Saturated fat and cholesterol are in foods that come from animals, such as meats, whole milk, egg yolks, butter, and cheese. Trans fat is found in fried foods and packaged foods, such as cookies, crackers, and chips.
- **Excess body weight**
- **Lack of physical activity**
- **Age**
  – men over age 45 and women over 55 are at higher risk.
- **Gender**
  – men are more prone to high cholesterol than women—until women reach 50 to 55 when naturally-occurring cholesterol levels in women increase.
- **Family history**
  – some people have a genetic predisposition to high cholesterol. Genes passed down from both sides of your families may cause your body to make too much or too little cholesterol.
- **Some diseases**
  – diabetes, thyroid disease, metabolic disease and others.
- **Cigarette smoking**
- **Certain medicines**
  – thiazide diuretics, beta-blockers, retinoids, estrogen and corticosteroids.

Prevention and Management

- **Get regular cholesterol screenings:**
  The first step in preventing high cholesterol and ultimately, heart disease, heart attack or stroke is to get a simple blood test to check your cholesterol levels. Healthy adults should have this test done every five years. If you are at increased risk for heart disease or if you are a man over 45 or a woman over 55, your doctor might have you tested more often.
- **Adopt a healthier lifestyle including:**
  – regular aerobic exercise
  – don't smoke
  – maintain a healthy weight
  – eat a nutritious diet low in saturated fat and cholesterol
- **Lower LDL levels**
  Clinical trials have demonstrated that lowering LDL cholesterol has many benefits and saves lives.
- **Take cholesterol medications, if prescribed by a health practitioner**
  Even after adopting a healthier lifestyle, your cholesterol level may not reach target and a medication may be required.

Risks of High Cholesterol

Cholesterol plays a big part in the development of atherosclerosis. Atherosclerosis is the buildup of fatty deposits including cholesterol, on the inner lining of arteries. This buildup (called plaque) may narrow the arteries causing a decrease in blood flow or a blood clot may develop which can clog or block the artery. As a result of this, cholesterol may increase the risk of heart disease, stroke, and other vascular diseases.

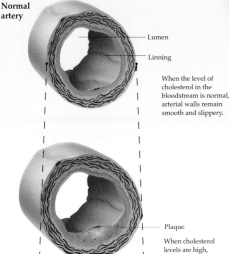

Normal artery

- Lumen
- Linning

When the level of cholesterol in the bloodstream is normal, arterial walls remain smooth and slippery.

- Plaque

When cholesterol levels are high, excess cholesterol can buildup on the walls of the arteries and may eventually reduce blood flow.

Clogged artery

- Ruptured plaque
- Blood clot

Plaque can rupture, resulting in a blood clot, which may cut off blood flow.

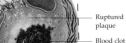

Advancing atherosclerosis

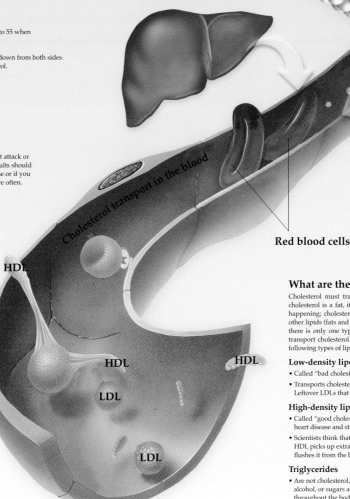

Phospholipid (other fats)

LIPOPROTEIN

Protein

Cholesterol

CHOLESTEROL MADE BY YOUR BODY (LIVER)

CHOLESTEROL FROM FOOD YOU EAT

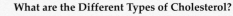

Cholesterol transport in the blood

Red blood cells

HDL
HDL
HDL
LDL
LDL

What are the Different Types of Cholesterol?

Cholesterol must travel through the bloodstream to get to your cells. Because cholesterol is a fat, it separates from blood like oil from water, to keep this from happening; cholesterol attaches to a protein. The combination of cholesterol and other lipids (fats and phyospholipds) with protein is called a lipoprotein. Although there is only one type of cholesterol, there are several types of lipoproteins that transport cholesterol. Blood tests for cholesterol generally provide results for the following types of lipoproteins:

Low-density lipoproteins (LDL) BAD CHOLESTEROL

- Called "bad cholesterol" because high levels can lead to heart disease and stroke.
- Transports cholesterol from you liver to the cells that need it. Leftover LDLs that are not needed release their cholesterol into the blood.

High-density lipoproteins (HDL) GOOD CHOLESTEROL

- Called "good cholesterol" because high levels reduce the risk for heart disease and stroke.
- Scientists think that HDL helps get rid of bad cholesterol in the blood. HDL picks up extra cholesterol and carries it to the liver, which then flushes it from the body.

Triglycerides

- Are not cholesterol, but are a different type of fat. Excess calories, alcohol, or sugars are converted into triglycerides and stored in fat cells throughout the body.
- High levels can raise the risk for heart disease.
- Are often part of a blood test doctors do to check cholesterol levels.

What Levels of Cholesterol are Healthy?

Knowing your cholesterol levels is an important part of understanding your own risk for heart disease. To determine how much cholesterol is in your body, your doctor will give you a blood test (also called a lipid profile or panel). Cholesterol levels are measured in milligrams (*mg*) of cholesterol per deciliter (dL) of blood in the United States and some other countries. The general guidelines below will help you understand your cholesterol test results.

TYPE	HEALTHY CHOLESTEROL LEVELS *	UNHEALTHY CHOLESTEROL LEVELS *
TOTAL CHOLESTEROL the level of all of the lipids (fats) in your blood, including LDL and HDL cholesterol	Less than 200 mg/dL Generally, a lower total cholesterol level is better.	200-239 mg/dL – borderline high 240 mg/dL and above – high A person with this level has more than twice the risk of heart disease as someone whose cholesterol is below 200 mg/dL.
LDL ("BAD" CHOLESTEROL)	Less than 70 md/dL – ideal for people at very high risk of heart disease and stroke. Less than 100 mg/dL – Lowest risk of heart attack and stroke.	100-129 mg/dL – near or above desirable 130-159 mg/dL – borderline high 160- 189 mg/dL – high 190 mg/dL and up - very high The more LDL there is in the blood, the greater the risk of heart disease. LDL cholesterol can build up on the walls of your arteries and over time may lead to heart attack or stroke.
HDL ("GOOD" CHOLESTEROL)	40 mg/dL or higher 60 mg/dL and above is considered protection against heart disease.	Less than 40 mg/dL (for men) Less than 50 mg/dL (for women) Low HDL cholesterol is a major risk factor for heart disease.
TRIGLYCERIDES	Less than 150 mg/dL (150 mg/dL is normal)	150-199 mg/dL – borderline high 200-499 mg/dL – hig 500 mg/dL and above – very high *Normal triglyceride levels vary by age and sex. High triglyceride levels in your blood can help clog arteries with plaque (cholesterol and fat buildup) and may raise the risk of heart attack and stroke. Above 600 mg/dL increases the risk for pancreatitis.

These levels should be used as a general guideline. Current recommendations might have changed and should be followed instead of what is stated here. Target levels also differ according to the number of risk factors you have for coronary artery disease. Please see your doctor to find out what your target level should be.

©2014 Wolters Kluwer

Understanding Colorectal Cancer

Transverse colon

Adenocarcinoma of colon

Circumferential carcinoma of transverse colon

Ascending colon

Cecum

Adenocarcinoma of jejunum

Colonic polyps

Descending colon

Vermiform appendix

Adenocarcinoma of rectosigmoid region

Rectum

Anus

Sigmoid colon

What is Colorectal Cancer? Cancer that begins in the colon is called colon cancer and cancer that begins in the rectum is called rectal cancer. Cancers affecting either of these organs is also called colorectal cancer.

Colorectal cancer occurs when some of the cells that line the colon or the rectum become abnormal and grow out of control. The abnormal growing cells create a tumor, which is the cancer.

Who is at Risk for Colorectal Cancer? Everybody is at risk for colorectal cancer. Colorectal cancer is the 2nd leading type of cancer causing deaths in the U.S.A. The majority of people who develop colorectal cancer have no known risk factors.

The exact cause of colorectal cancer is not yet known. Below are some factors that could increase a person's risk of developing this disease.

- **Age -** The disease is more common in people over 50. The chance of getting colorectal cancer increases with each decade of life. However, it has also been detected in younger people.
- **Gender -** Overall the risks are equal, but women have a higher risk for colon cancer and men are more likely to develop rectal cancer.
- **Polyps -** Begin as non-cancerous growths on the inner wall of the colon or rectum; this is fairly common in people over 50 years of age. Adenomas are one type of non-cancerous polyps that can mutate and are the potential precursors of colon and rectal cancer.
- **Personal history -** Research shows that women who have a history of ovarian or uterine cancer have a slight increased risk of developing colorectal cancer. In addition, people who have Ulcerative colitis or Crohn's disease also are at higher risk.
- **Family history -** Parents, siblings, and children of a person who has had colorectal cancer are more likely to develop the disease themselves. A family history of familial polyposis, adenomatous polyps, or hereditary polyp syndrome also increases the risk.
- **Diet -** A diet high in fat and calories and low in fiber may be linked to a greater risk.
- **Lifestyle factors -** Alcohol, smoking, lack of exercise, and overweight status are additional risk factors.
- **Diabetes -** Diabetics have a 30-40% increased risk.

Signs & Symptoms

Colorectal cancer may not cause any symptoms in early stages. However the following signs should raise suspicion:

- Change in bowel habits: Diarrhea or constipation or a change in the consistency of stool
- Narrow, pencil-thin stools
- Rectal bleed or blood in stool
- Persistent abdominal discomfort such as gas, pain or cramps
- Feeling bowel does not empty completely
- Unexplained weight loss
- Constant fatigue

Screening tests

- **Fecal Occult Blood Test (FOBT) -** Checks for hidden blood in the stool.
- **Sigmoidoscopy -** Sigmoidoscope is a long, flexible tube with a tiny video camera at the tip that is inserted into the rectum to allow the doctor to view the lower part of the colon – the rectum, the descending colon, and the sigmoid colon.
- **Colonoscopy -** Colonoscope is a long, flexible tube with a tiny video camera at the tip that is inserted into the rectum to allow the doctor to view the inside of the entire colon. The doctor may also biopsy the tissue and remove polyps during a colonoscopy.
- **Barium enema -** Chalky white liquid called barium is released into the colon (through the rectum) and then an X-ray is performed.
- **Digital rectal exam**

Diagnostic tests

If the screening tests or symptoms indicate the possibility of colorectal cancer, patients will undergo a diagnostic workup. These will help determine if colorectal cancer is present and the stage of the disease. Tests may include:

- **Medical history**
- **Physical exam**
- **Blood tests**
- **Biopsy -** abnormal tissue is removed and examined during a screening test to check for cancer cells.
- **Imaging Tests**
- **Ultrasound**
- **Computed tomography (CT)**
- **Magnetic resonance imaging (MRI)**
- **Chest X-ray** (to see if the cancer has spread to the lungs)

Treatments

Choice of treatment(s) depends on the location of the tumor (colon or rectum) and the stage of the disease. Common types of treatments include:

- **Surgery -** This is the most common treatment. It is used for removal of polyps and tumors and to check for the spread of the disease. Common types include laparoscopy and open surgery. After removal of part of the colon or rectum, the healthy parts are usually reconnected. When reconnection is not possible, a colostomy may be performed.
- **Chemotherapy -** Drug therapy that prevents the spread of cancer cells.
- **Radiation Therapy -** Also known as Radiotherapy, uses high energy-rays to kill cancer cells.
- **Biological Therapy -** Patients receive a monoclonal antibody through a vein which binds to colorectal cancer cells, interfering with their cell growth and spread in the body.

The Stages of Cancer

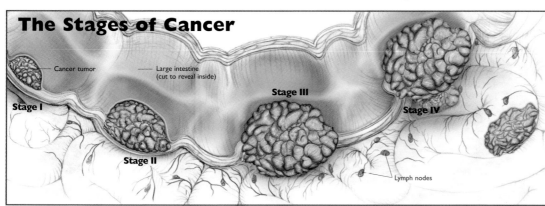

Cancer tumor

Large intestine (cut to reveal inside)

Stage III

Stage I

Stage IV

Stage II

Lymph nodes

The earlier cancer is found and treated, the better the chances of getting well. The diagnosis of cancer is made by a microscopic test (biopsy) of a piece of tissue. Medical imaging techniques are used to measure how much the cancer has spread (grown) – this is known as staging.
The doctors often decide on the treatment based on the stage of cancer.

Doctors identify the stages of cancer as follows:

Stage I: The cancer has grown into the inner wall of the colon or rectum. The tumor has not yet reached the outer wall of the colon or extended outside the colon. Dukes' A is another name for Stage I colorectal cancer.

Stage II: The tumor extends more deeply into or through the wall of the colon or rectum. It may have invaded nearby tissue, but cancer cells have not yet spread to the lymph nodes. Dukes' B is another name for Stage II colorectal cancer.

Stage III: The cancer has spread to nearby lymph nodes, but not to other parts of the body. Dukes' C is another name for Stage III colorectal cancer.

Stage IV: The cancer has spread to other parts of the body, such as the liver or lungs. Dukes' D is another name for Stage IV colorectal cancer.

©2014 Wolters Kluwer

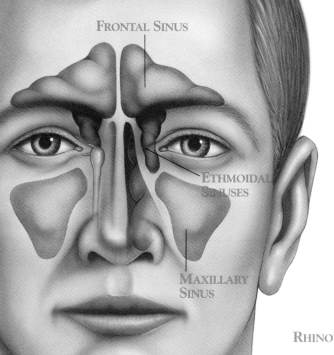

FRONTAL SINUS

ETHMOIDAL SINUSES

MAXILLARY SINUS

COMMON COLD IS A VIRAL INFECTION OF THE UPPER RESPIRATORY TRACT (NOSE AND THROAT), WHICH CAUSES THE MUCUS MEMBRANES OF THE HEAD AND THROAT TO BECOME INFLAMED. USUALLY COLDS LAST FROM 3 – 7 DAYS ALTHOUGH SOME OF THE SYMPTOMS CAN LAST FOR 2 WEEKS. RARELY, A BACTERIAL INFECTION MAY COMPLICATE A COLD CAUSED BY A VIRUS.

RHINOVIRUS

HEADACHE

SINUS PAIN

RUNNY OR STUFFY NOSE

COUGHING OR SORE THROAT

CAUSES AND RISK FACTORS

Most colds are caused by the rhinovirus and are highly contagious (especially the first 2 - 4 days). The virus enters the body through the mouth or nose.

Colds can be caught by:

- Inhaling the droplets of the virus from someone who is sick as they cough, sneeze or talk.
- Having direct physical contact with someone who has a cold; touching objects that they have touched and then touching your own eyes, nose, or mouth can transfer the virus into your system.

Risk Factors

- Age: Infants and younger children are more susceptible to colds because of their immature immune systems and their close contact with other children. As the immune system develops over time, the frequency of colds diminishes.
- Season: Children and adults are more likely to catch colds in the fall and winter (or during rainy seasons) when more time is spent indoors.
- Additionally: Fatigue, stress, and allergies that have nose or throat symptoms can increase the risk of getting a cold.

SIGNS AND SYMPTOMS

The symptoms you experience during a cold are due to inflammation. When foreign microorganisms such as viruses enter the body, your body's defenses react with an inflammatory response; this response is characterized by redness, heat, swelling, and pain. As the body attacks and breaks down the cold virus, the resulting debris is blown out from the nose or coughed up from the air passages in the lungs.

The symptoms resulting from this process can include:

- Runny or stuffy nose
- Sneezing
- Sore or tickly throat
- Watery eyes
- Coughing
- Headache
- Sinus pain or teeth pain (viral sinusitis can occur with a cold)
- Muscle aches
- Mild fever
- Fatigue
- Decreased appetite

COMPLICATIONS OF THE COMMON COLD

When you have a cold, asthma may become worse, including wheezing.

You may also acquire bacterial infections such as:

- Sinusitis
- Bronchitis
- Ear Infections (usually in children)
- Pneumonia

TREATMENT AND MANAGEMENT

There is no cure for the common cold, but there are things you can do to make yourself more comfortable, including:

- Drink plenty of liquids.
- Eat chicken soup.
- Rest and consider staying home while you are sick.
- Gargle with warm salt water.
- Use nasal saline or a Neti pot.
- Use a humidifier - remember to change the water daily.
- For adults and children, pain relievers such as acetaminophen or ibuprofen can help reduce muscle aches or fever.
- Always talk to your doctor before giving cold medicine to children 6 years of age and younger.

It is important to note that antibiotics are not effective against viral infections such as the common cold. Antibiotics work only against bacterial infections.

When to suspect a bacterial infection or complications from a cold and seek medical help:

- If symptoms do not improve or they worsen after 7 – 10 days.
- If you have difficulty breathing.
- If you have persistent fever.

TO PREVENT GETTING THE COLD VIRUS...

Keep your hands away from your face and eyes.

Wash your hands frequently with soap and water for 15 – 30 seconds. If a sink is not available, alcohol-based rubs can be used as an alternative.

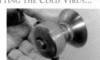

Keep surfaces and objects (countertops, door knobs, toys, etc.) that can be exposed to the virus clean.

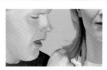

Avoid close contact with people who have a cold.

TO PREVENT SPREADING THE COLD VIRUS...

Avoid close contact with others and don't share utensils or drinking glasses.

Cover your mouth and nose with a tissue when coughing or sneezing. If there is no tissue available, cough or sneeze into your elbow rather than your hands.

©2014 Wolters Kluwer

43

Understanding Depression

What Is Depression?

Depression is a serious medical condition that affects thoughts, moods, feelings, behavior, and physical health. There are different types of depressions, the most common is Major Depressive Disorder. Major Depressive Disorder and other types of serious depressions are "long-lasting" and get in the way of a person's ability to work, study, sleep, and eat.

Signs and Symptoms of Major Depression

A person may have depression if five or more of the following symptoms are present for more than two weeks at any one time; this should be reported to a healthcare provider.

- Loss of interest or enjoyment in normal daily activities
- Persistent sad, anxious, or hopeless mood
- Irritability or nervousness
- Feelings of guilt, fear, or worthlessness
- Significant weight loss or gain due to appetite change
- Overtiredness and/or decreased energy
- Unable to sleep or too much sleep
- Unexplained crying spells
- Difficulty concentrating, remembering, and/or making decisions
- Little or no interest in companionship or sex
- Thoughts of death or suicide

If thoughts of suicide exist, or if symptoms get in the way of daily activities, one should seek treatment right away.

Who is at Risk for Depression?

Although depression can be triggered by personal problems, other factors also affect who becomes depressed. Often, a combination of risk factors are involved.

- **Heredity:** Some types of depression run in families. However, not everyone with a family history of depression will develop the disorder.
- **Gender:** Twice as many women as men experience depression.
- **Hormonal Changes:** Changing hormone levels, as in the post-partum period, may cause depression.
- **Alcohol and Drug Abuse**
- **Medications:** Certain drugs can cause depression, so it is important for patients to provide a complete list of medications to their health care provider.
- **Physical Disease:** Illnesses such as stroke, heart attack, cancer, Parkinson's disease, hormonal disorders and viral infections can cause depression.
- **Stress:** Traumatic experiences, such as the loss of a love one, can trigger depression.

Areas of the Brain Affected by Depression

Some areas of the brain are underactive in depression, while other areas are over-active. These changes contribute to the emotional and physical symptoms of depression.

Thalamus
Controls a person's degree of arousal and awareness, including sleep and hypervigilance. It stimulates the amygdala. The thalamus is highly active in people with depression.

Hypothalamus
Produces the neurotransmitters that are involved in mood and emotional expressions. Serotonin pathways in the hypothalamus help regulate mood and appetite while norepinephrine pathways help regulate emotions and energy level.

Amygdala
Responsible for negative feelings; it is highly active in people with depression.

Anterior cingulate cortex
Helps associate smells and sights with pleasant memories. It also has a role in emotional response to pain and the regulation of anger. This area is highly active in people with depression.

Prefrontal cortex
Involved in complex thinking, personality, and social behavior. Norepinephrine and serotonin are two neurotransmitters that affect mood in this part of the brain.
Norepinephrine pathways impact attention span, concentration, memory, and information processing. There is decreased activity in the prefrontal cortex in depression.

The Limbic System

Regulates emotions, instincts, motivations and sexual drive. It also plays a role in the body's response to stress. Any disturbances to the limbic system can affect mood and behavior.

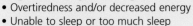

Hippocampus
Amygdala
Fornix
Thalamus
Mamillary body

The Role of Neurotransmitters

Neurotransmitters are chemicals that carry messages between the nerve cells (neurons); these affect behavior, mood, and thought. Depression is related to these chemical imbalances in the brain.

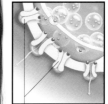

Abnormal

With low levels of norepinephrine and serotonin neurotransmitters, membrane channels do not open; as a result, nerve messages are not passed on, and areas of the brain that affect emotions may not receive stimulation. This process may result in depression.

Closed membrane channels seen on a neuron affected by depression

Normal

Opened membrane channels seen on a neuron not affected by depression

Other Types of Depression

Dysthymic Disorder (Dysthymia)

Dysthymic disorder is a milder, more chronic form of depression compared to major depressive disorder. A person may feel depressed one day and normal on another day. Although the symptoms are not as disabling, having dysthymia increases the risk of developing major depression.

Bipolar Disorder (Manic-Depressive Illness)

Bipolar disorder is described as recurring cycles of intense moods. A person may experience recurrent "high" moods (mania), very "low" moods (depression), or switching between these highs and lows. During the "highs", one may be too confident, very talkative, energetic, impulsive and take high risks. One may also get very little sleep, be very irritable, and make poor decisions. During the "lows", one may appear depressed and unable to concentrate.

Suicide

People who are depressed are at higher risk for suicide. If a person feels life is not worth living, especially if one is thinking about ending his/her life, seek treatment immediately.

Any threat of suicide should be taken seriously. Contact a mental health professional or suicide hotline immediately if you experience any of the following danger signs.

- Pacing, nervous behavior, frequent mood changes (this symptom by itself is not an emergency or suggestive of being suicidal)
- Actions or threats of physical harm or violence
- Threats or talking of death or suicide
- Withdrawal from activities and relationships (by itself, this is not an emergency)
- Giving away prized possessions or saying goodbye to friends
- A sudden brightening of mood after a period of severe depression
- Unusually risky behavior

Treatment

Depression can almost always be treated effectively. Certain medications and medical conditions can also cause the same symptoms as depression; the diagnosis of depression must be made by a health professional. If depression is diagnosed, treatment can include one or more of the following:

Antidepressants

These medications rebalance key chemicals, neurotransmitters, in the brain and take time to work. Neurotransmitters are required for the brain to function normally. A variety of antidepressants may be tried before finding the treatment that may work best for you.

Counseling (Psychotherapy)

Counseling involves talking with a trained mental health professional. It helps people gain insight into their feelings and learn how to deal with them, change behaviors, and resolve problems.

Mood Stabilizers

These medications help soothe mood swings. Many people with bipolar disorder may take mood stabilizers to "even out" their moods.

Alternative Therapies

- **Herbal therapy** may have a beneficial effect on mild cases of depression. Talk to your healthcare provider before taking any herbal or dietary supplement.
- **Regular Exercise** can ease the symptoms of mild depression. Research indicates that physical activity has a positive effect on brain chemicals, which can improve mood and sense of well being.

©2014 Wolters Kluwer

Understanding Diabetes

44

What Is Diabetes?

Diabetes mellitus is the name for a group of chronic diseases that affect the way the body uses food to make the energy necessary for life. Diabetes is a disruption of carbohydrate (sugar and starch) metabolism, but it also affects fat and protein metabolism. This leads to hyperglycemia (increased blood glucose). High blood glucose for an extended period of time can result in damage to various parts of the body. There are two main forms of diabetes, Type 1 (insulin-dependent or juvenile) and Type 2 (non-insulin-dependent or adult-onset). Some secondary forms also exist, caused by conditions such as pancreatic disease, pregnancy (gestational diabetes mellitus), hormonal or genetic problems, and certain drugs.

Brain

Lung

Heart

Liver

Stomach

Pancreas

Kidney

Large intestine

Small intestine

Type 1 Diabetes

Type 1 diabetes is a disease in which the pancreas produces little or no insulin. Insulin is needed to transport glucose into the cells for use as energy and storage as glycogen (sugar). It also stimulates protein synthesis and free fatty acid storage in the fat deposits. When a person lacks sufficient insulin, body tissues have less access to essential nutrients for fuel and storage. Type 1 diabetes usually develops before age 30, although it may strike at any age.

Type 2 Diabetes

In Type 2 diabetes, the pancreas produces some insulin, but it is either too little or is not effective. Also, insulin receptors that control the transport of glucose into cells may not work properly (insulin resistance) or are reduced in number. The more common form of diabetes, Type 2 typically develops in adults over age 40, but it can appear earlier. Type 2 diabetes may also develop as a consequence of obesity.

Potential Complications of Diabetes:

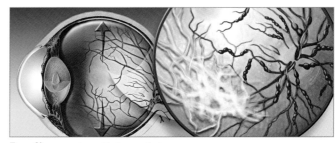

Stroke: Causing loss of neurologic function, leading to numbness, weakness, difficulty with speech, coordination, or walking.

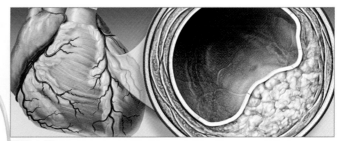

Eye disease: Causing blind spots or blindness.

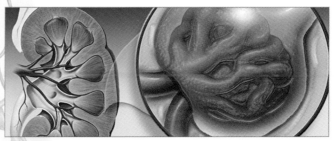

Heart disease: Causing heart attacks and congestive heart failure.

Kidney disease: Causing kidney failure.

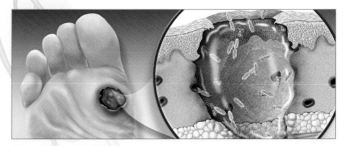

Circulatory problems: Causing sores that do not heal well. In extreme situations, gangrene can develop and can lead to amputations.

What Are the Symptoms of Diabetes?

Patients with **Type 1 diabetes** usually report rapidly developing symptoms. With **Type 2 diabetes**, symptoms usually develop gradually and may not appear until many years after the onset of the disease.

Some of the symptoms for Type 1 or Type 2 diabetes are included in the following list.

- Sudden weight loss
- Frequent urination
- Extreme hunger
- Excessive thirst
- Blurred vision
- Dry, itchy skin
- More infections than usual
- Numbness in feet, hands
- Slow-healing cuts or sores
- Fatigue or tiredness
- No symptoms

What Are the Long-Term Health Problems?

High blood glucose levels caused by diabetes may damage small and large blood vessels and nerves. Diabetes may also lower the body's ability to fight infection. Because of these changes, people with diabetes are more likely to have serious eye problems, kidney disease, heart attacks, strokes, high blood pressure, circulatory problems, numbness of the feet, sexual problems, and infections. Patients with diabetes should be checked regularly for signs of these complications, many of which can be reduced or delayed with good blood glucose control and regular medical care.

©2014 Wolters Kluwer

Diseases of the Digestive System

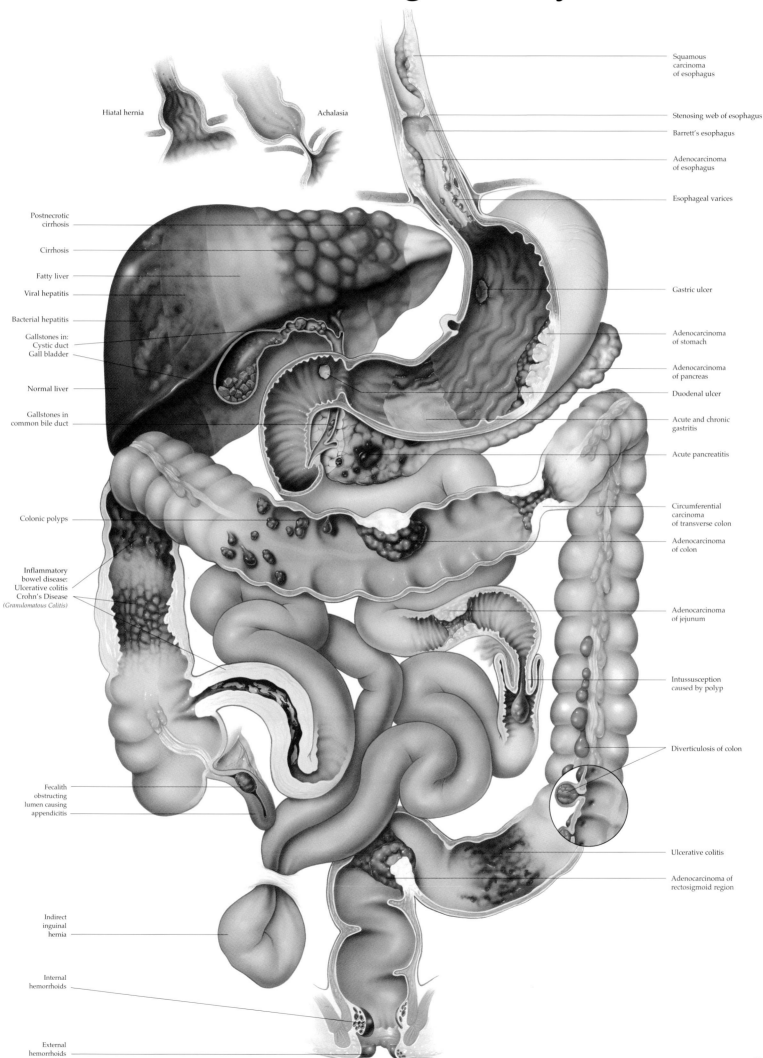

45

Hiatal hernia

Achalasia

Squamous carcinoma of esophagus

Stenosing web of esophagus

Barrett's esophagus

Adenocarcinoma of esophagus

Esophageal varices

Postnecrotic cirrhosis

Cirrhosis

Fatty liver

Viral hepatitis

Bacterial hepatitis

Gallstones in: Cystic duct Gall bladder

Normal liver

Gallstones in common bile duct

Gastric ulcer

Adenocarcinoma of stomach

Adenocarcinoma of pancreas

Duodenal ulcer

Acute and chronic gastritis

Acute pancreatitis

Colonic polyps

Circumferential carcinoma of transverse colon

Adenocarcinoma of colon

Inflammatory bowel disease: Ulcerative colitis Crohn's Disease *(Granulomatous Colitis)*

Adenocarcinoma of jejunum

Intussusception caused by polyp

Diverticulosis of colon

Fecalith obstructing lumen causing appendicitis

Ulcerative colitis

Adenocarcinoma of rectosigmoid region

Indirect inguinal hernia

Internal hemorrhoids

External hemorrhoids

©2014 Wolters Kluwer

46

Gastroesophageal Disorders and Digestive Anatomy

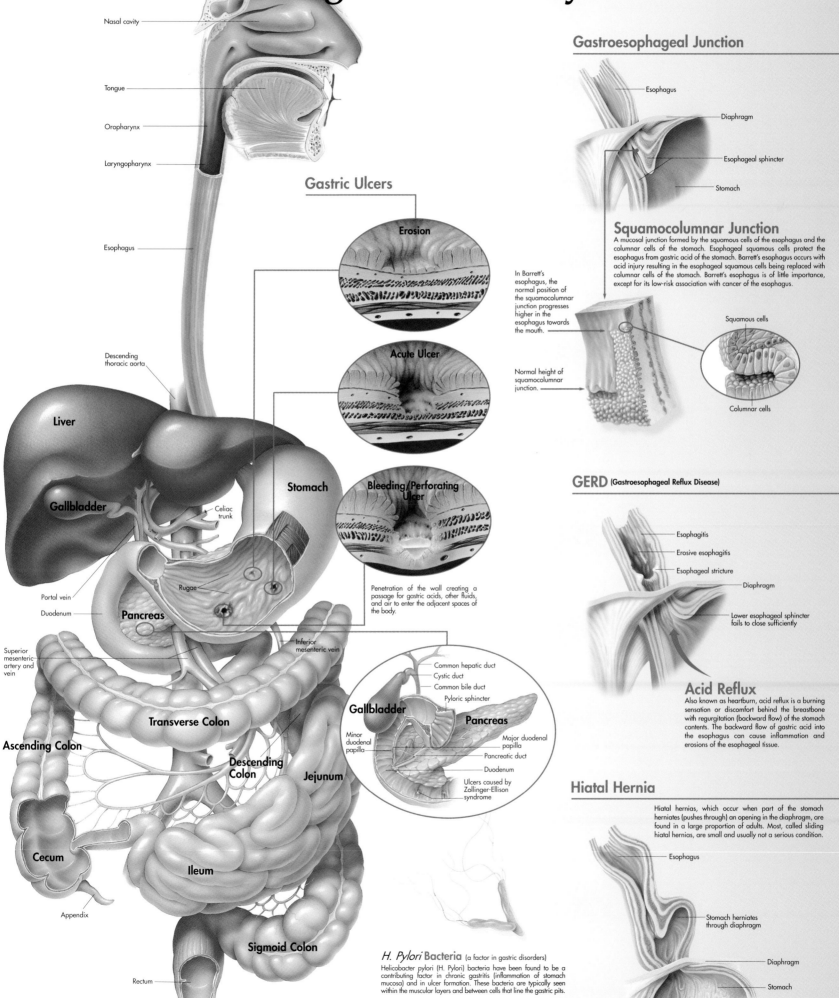

Nasal cavity

Tongue

Oropharynx

Laryngopharynx

Esophagus

Descending thoracic aorta

Liver

Gallbladder

Portal vein

Duodenum

Pancreas

Superior mesenteric artery and vein

Ascending Colon

Transverse Colon

Descending Colon

Jejunum

Cecum

Ileum

Appendix

Sigmoid Colon

Rectum

Anus

Celiac trunk

Rugae

Inferior mesenteric vein

Stomach

Gastric Ulcers

Erosion

Acute Ulcer

Bleeding/Perforating Ulcer

Penetration of the wall creating a passage for gastric acids, other fluids, and air to enter the adjacent spaces of the body.

In Barrett's esophagus, the normal position of the squamocolumnar junction progresses higher in the esophagus towards the mouth.

Normal height of squamocolumnar junction.

Common hepatic duct
Cystic duct
Common bile duct
Pyloric sphincter

Gallbladder

Pancreas

Minor duodenal papilla

Major duodenal papilla
Pancreatic duct
Duodenum
Ulcers caused by Zollinger-Ellison syndrome

H. Pylori Bacteria (a factor in gastric disorders)
Helicobacter pylori (H. Pylori) bacteria have been found to be a contributing factor in chronic gastritis (inflammation of stomach mucosa) and in ulcer formation. These bacteria are typically seen within the muscular layers and between cells that line the gastric pits.

Gastroesophageal Junction

Esophagus
Diaphragm
Esophageal sphincter
Stomach

Squamocolumnar Junction
A mucosal junction formed by the squamous cells of the esophagus and the columnar cells of the stomach. Esophageal squamous cells protect the esophagus from gastric acid of the stomach. Barrett's esophagus occurs with acid injury resulting in the esophageal squamous cells being replaced with columnar cells of the stomach. Barrett's esophagus is of little importance, except for its low-risk association with cancer of the esophagus.

Squamous cells

Columnar cells

GERD (Gastroesophageal Reflux Disease)

Esophagitis
Erosive esophagitis
Esophageal stricture
Diaphragm
Lower esophageal sphincter fails to close sufficiently

Acid Reflux
Also known as heartburn, acid reflux is a burning sensation or discomfort behind the breastbone with regurgitation (backward flow) of the stomach contents. The backward flow of gastric acid into the esophagus can cause inflammation and erosions of the esophageal tissue.

Hiatal Hernia

Hiatal hernias, which occur when part of the stomach herniates (pushes through) an opening in the diaphragm, are found in a large proportion of adults. Most, called sliding hiatal hernias, are small and usually not a serious condition.

Esophagus

Stomach herniates through diaphragm

Diaphragm

Stomach

©2014 Wolters Kluwer

Understanding Influenza

47

What Is Influenza?

Influenza, also known as the flu, is caused by the influenza virus. It is a contagious infection of the nose, throat, and lungs.

Influenza virus spreads in the little drops that spray out of an infected person's mouth and nose when he sneezes, coughs, laughs, or even talks.

When someone else breathes in these drops or gets them on his hands and then touches his own mouth or nose, the virus can enter his body .

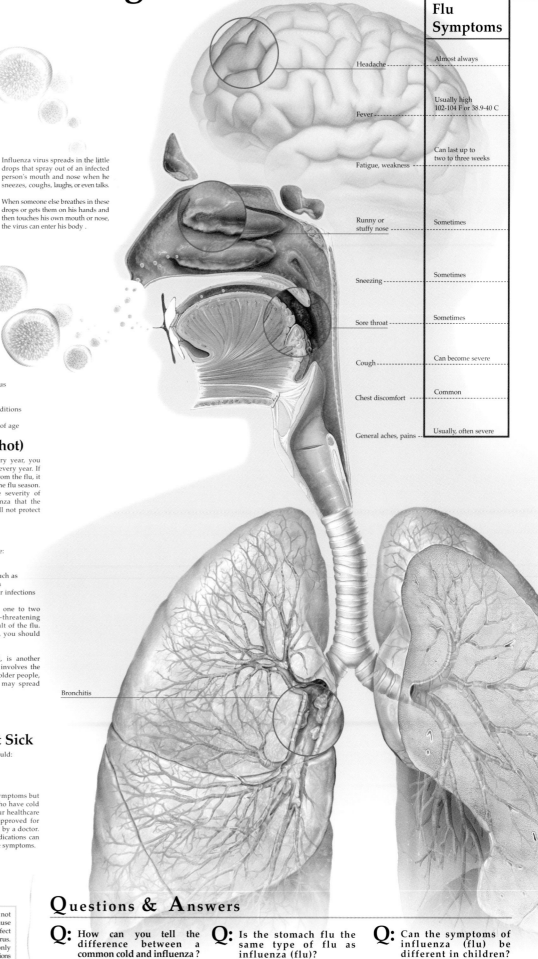

Flu Symptoms

Headache	Almost always
Fever	Usually high 102-104 F or 38.9-40 C
Fatigue, weakness	Can last up to two to three weeks
Runny or stuffy nose	Sometimes
Sneezing	Sometimes
Sore throat	Sometimes
Cough	Can become severe
Chest discomfort	Common
General aches, pains	Usually, often severe

Prevention

Ways to Help Prevent Influenza

Avoid touching your eyes, nose, and mouth.

Wash your hands with soap and water frequently.

Get a vaccination (flu shot) every year before the start of the flu season. *Note: The vaccine does not cause the flu.*

Ways to Help Prevent the Spread of Influenza

Stay home when you are sick.

Avoid close contact with others.

Cover your mouth and nose with a tissue when coughing or sneezing.

Special Risk Factors

Certain people have an increased risk of serious complications from influenza:
• People age 65 years and older
• People of any age with chronic medical conditions
• Pregnant women
• Children between 6 months and 23 months of age

Flu Vaccination (Flu Shot)

Because the influenza virus is different every year, you should protect yourself by getting a flu shot every year. If you are at high risk for major complications from the flu, it is especially important to get the shot before the flu season. The influenza vaccine may also lessen the severity of symptoms related to other forms of influenza that the vaccine is unable to prevent. The flu shot will not protect you from the common cold.

Complications

The complications caused by influenza include:
• Bacterial pneumonia
• Dehydration
• Worsening of chronic medical conditions, such as congestive heart failure, asthma, or diabetes
• Children may develop sinus problems or ear infections

Most people who get influenza recover in one to two weeks, but some people develop life-threatening complications (such as pneumonia) as a result of the flu. If your flu symptoms are unusually severe , you should seek medical help immediately.

Bronchitis, or inflammation of the bronchi, is another complication of influenza. In most cases, it involves the large and medium-sized bronchi. In children, older people, and those with lung disease, the infection may spread and inflame the bronchioles or lung tissue.

Bronchitis

What to Do If You Get Sick

If you develop an influenza infection, you should:
• Get plenty of rest
• Drink plenty of liquids
• Avoid using alcohol and tobacco

You can also take medications to relieve flu symptoms but never give aspirin to children or teenagers who have cold or flu symptoms without first speaking to your healthcare provider. Antiviral medications have been approved for treatment of influenza but must be prescribed by a doctor. There is no cure for the flu. The antiviral medications can help reduce the severity and the duration of the symptoms.

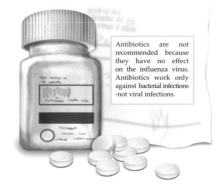

Antibiotics are not recommended because they have no effect on the influenza virus. Antibiotics work only against bacterial infections -not viral infections.

Questions & Answers

Q: How can you tell the difference between a common cold and influenza ?

A: Although flu and cold symptoms can be similar, the intensity and duration are different. The symptoms of a cold may come on gradually and are milder than the symptoms of the flu. Flu symptoms are more severe and tend to come on immediately and take longer to recover.

Q: Is the stomach flu the same type of flu as influenza (flu)?

A: No. Some people use the term "stomach flu" to describe certain common illnesses that can cause nausea, vomiting, or diarrhea. Although these symptoms can sometimes be related to the flu (more commonly in children), these problems are rarely symptoms of influenza.

Q: Can the symptoms of influenza (flu) be different in children?

A: Yes. Although flu symptoms for children and adults might be similar, children might have other symptoms such as nausea, vomiting and/or diarrhea. Children are at a higher risk of complications from the flu. If a child's symptoms worsen, call your doctor.

©2014 Wolters Kluwer

48

Understanding Lung Cancer

Lung cancer is the rapid growth of abnormal (malignant) cells that originate from a lung cell. Like any cancer it can invade nearby tissues and may spread (metastasize) to other areas of the body.

Trachea

Lymph nodes

Metastasis to paratracheal lymph nodes

Bronchus

Tumor projecting into bronchi

Metastasis to carinal lymph nodes

LEFT UPPER LOBE

Tumor projecting into bronchi

LEFT LOWER LOBE

APPROXIMATELY 90% OF LUNG CANCER DEATHS ARE RELATED TO SMOKING

There are 2 Major Types of Lung Cancer:
Non-Small Cell Lung Cancer and Small Cell Lung Cancer

Non-small cell lung cancer (NSCLC) is more common than small cell lung cancer, accounting for about 85% of all lung cancers; it generally grows and spreads more slowly. The three most common types of non-small cell lung cancer are:

1. **Adenocarcinoma** is the most common sub-type of NSCLC. It is usually found in the outer part of the lung.
2. **Squamous cell carcinoma** are tumors originating in the lining of the bronchus.
3. **Large cell carcinoma** can develop in any part of the lung.

NSCLC is staged according to the size of the tumor, the level of lymph node involvement, and whether the cancer has spread. Stages include:

Stage 0	Cancer is limited to the lining of the air passages and has not yet invaded the lung tissue.
Stage I	Cancer has invaded the underlying lung tissue, but has not yet spread to the lymph nodes.
Stage II	Cancer has spread to the neighboring lymph nodes.
Stage III	Cancer has spread from the lung to either the lymph nodes in the center of the chest or the collarbone area. The cancer may have spread locally to areas such as the heart, blood vessels, trachea, and esophagus.
Stage IV	Cancer has spread to other parts of the body, such as the liver, bones, or brain.

Small cell lung cancer (SCLC), also known as oat cell cancer, is the less common form of lung cancer. It is a very fast-growing lung cancer and can rapidly spread to other parts of the body.

SCLC is staged differently from non-small cell types. Rather than using numbers, it is classified as either limited or extensive.

Limited	Cancer is confined to one lung and to its neighboring lymph nodes.
Extensive	Cancer has spread beyond one lung and nearby lymph nodes; it may have invaded both lungs, more remote lymph nodes, or other organs.

How is Lung Cancer Diagnosed?
The tests used to diagnose whether a patient has lung cancer varies depending on the patient's symptoms.

Chest X-Ray – Most patients may first undergo this test to see if there are any abnormalities.

Chest CT Scan – If an abnormality is discovered in the chest x-ray, a computerized tomography (CT) scan is performed to provide a series of detailed pictures taken from different angles.

Biopsy – There are several different types of biopsy procedures. The choice of procedure, which may involve surgery, will depend on how big the tumor is, where it is located, and if it has spread outside the lung.

Sputum Cytology – A sample of phlegm is examined under a microscope to search for cancer cells.

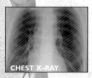
CHEST X-RAY

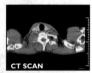
CT SCAN

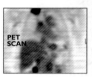
PET SCAN

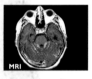
MRI

How is Lung Cancer Staged?
If cancer is diagnosed, more tests are done so the physician can plan the best treatment. The type of treatment recommended will depend on the stage of the cancer. The following tests can help discover the stage (extent) of the cancer:

Positron Emission Tomography (PET) scan – A small amount of radioactive glucose (sugar) is injected into a vein of a patient, the cancer cells take up the radioactive glucose and a special camera makes computerized pictures highlighting potential cancer cells.

PET/CT Scan – PET scan information is combined with the anatomical information from a CT scan to reliably determine whether an abnormal growth is cancerous or benign (non-cancerous).

Magnetic Resonance Imaging (MRI) of the Brain – A powerful magnet linked to a computer produces detailed images of the areas inside the brain, which can help to determine if lung cancer has spread to the brain.

Mediastinoscopy/ Mediastinotomy – A lighted instrument (scope) is inserted into the chest to examine the lymph nodes which can be the first place for lung cancer to spread.

Risk Factors
Smoking cigarettes is by far the most common cause of lung cancer.
• Smoking cigarettes, cigars, and pipes – 90% of patients that develop lung cancer are current or ex-smokers.

Less common risk factors include:
• Having previous lung diseases, such as tuberculosis (TB) and emphysema
• Personal history – a person with a history of lung cancer is more likely to develop it again than someone who has never had the disease
• Heredity – genetics seem to play a role in who develops lung cancer
• Exposure to secondhand smoke
• Exposure to radon, a naturally occurring radioactive gas in soil and rock which may also be found homes and buildings
• Exposure to asbestos, a group of naturally occurring fibrous minerals that are used in some industries
• Pollution

Signs and Symptoms
• **Cough that does not go away**
• **Constant chest pain**
• **Coughing up blood**
• **Shortness of breath, wheezing, or hoarseness**
• **Swelling of the neck and face**
• **Loss of appetite and/or weight**
• **Fatigue**

If lung cancer has spread to other organs (metastasized), signs may include headaches, visual changes, stroke-like symptoms (if cancer has spread to the brain), and bone pain (if the cancer has spread to the bones).

Treatment Options
Treatment depends on a number of factors including the type of lung cancer, the size/location/stage of the tumor, and the general health and pulmonary function of the patient. Many different types of treatments or combination of treatments may be used, such as:

Surgical Resection – A portion of the lung containing the tumor is removed. Depending on the case, the surgeon may remove only a small portion, the entire lobe (lobectomy), or the entire lung (pneumonectomy). Lymph nodes are also sampled at the time of surgery. Lobectomy is the most widely used surgical procedure for lung cancer.

Chemotherapy – The use of anticancer drugs that kill cancer cells throughout the body.

Radiation therapy – The use of high-energy rays to kill cancer cells. This therapy is directed to specific site and affects the cancer cells only in that area.

Endobronchial Therapy – A group of therapies used to remove tumors that are accessible inside the lung airway and causing a blockage of the airway (resulting in shortness of breath). They are used for palliative therapy to relieve symptoms, not to cure the cancer.

How can Lung Cancer be Prevented?
• **Don't smoke** – If you do smoke, quit. If you stop smoking, the risk of lung cancer decreases each year as normal cells replace abnormal cells. After 10 years, the risk drops to a level that is one-third to one-half of the risk of people who continue to smoke.
• **Avoid secondhand smoke**
• **Test your home for radon**
• **Avoid carcinogens** - People who are exposed to large amounts of asbestos should use protective equipment.

©2014 Wolters Kluwer

Diseases of the Lung

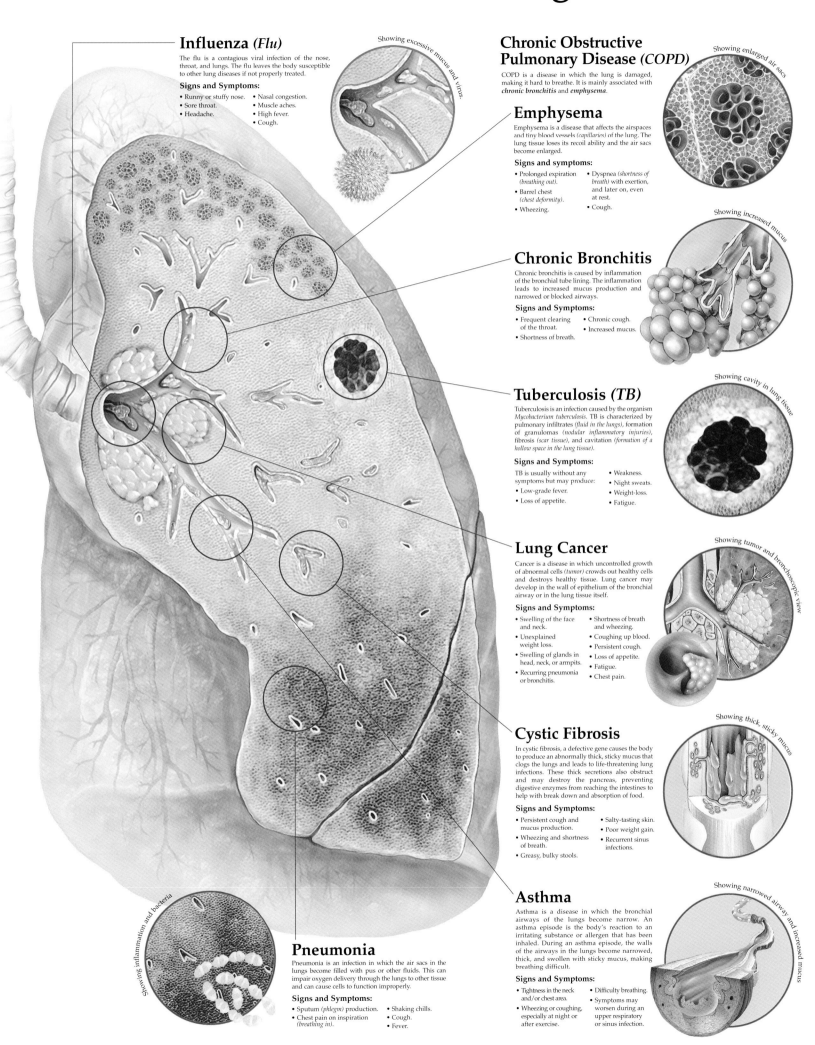

49

Influenza (Flu)

The flu is a contagious viral infection of the nose, throat, and lungs. The flu leaves the body susceptible to other lung diseases if not properly treated.

Signs and Symptoms:

- Runny or stuffy nose.
- Sore throat.
- Headache.
- Nasal congestion.
- Muscle aches.
- High fever.
- Cough.

Showing excessive mucus and virus.

Chronic Obstructive Pulmonary Disease (COPD)

COPD is a disease in which the lung is damaged, making it hard to breathe. It is mainly associated with *chronic bronchitis* and *emphysema*.

Emphysema

Emphysema is a disease that affects the airspaces and tiny blood vessels (*capillaries*) of the lung. The lung tissue loses its recoil ability and the air sacs become enlarged.

Signs and symptoms:

- Prolonged expiration (*breathing out*).
- Barrel chest (*chest deformity*).
- Wheezing.
- Dyspnea (*shortness of breath*) with exertion, and later on, even at rest.
- Cough.

Showing enlarged air sacs

Chronic Bronchitis

Chronic bronchitis is caused by inflammation of the bronchial tube lining. The inflammation leads to increased mucus production and narrowed or blocked airways.

Signs and Symptoms:

- Frequent clearing of the throat.
- Shortness of breath.
- Chronic cough.
- Increased mucus.

Showing increased mucus

Tuberculosis (TB)

Tuberculosis is an infection caused by the organism *Mycobacterium tuberculosis*. TB is characterized by pulmonary infiltrates (*fluid in the lungs*), formation of granulomas (*nodular inflammatory injuries*), fibrosis (*scar tissue*), and cavitation (*formation of a hollow space in the lung tissue*).

Signs and Symptoms:

TB is usually without any symptoms but may produce:
- Low-grade fever.
- Loss of appetite.
- Weakness.
- Night sweats.
- Weight-loss.
- Fatigue.

Showing cavity in lung tissue

Lung Cancer

Cancer is a disease in which uncontrolled growth of abnormal cells (*tumor*) crowds out healthy cells and destroys healthy tissue. Lung cancer may develop in the wall of epithelium of the bronchial airway or in the lung tissue itself.

Signs and Symptoms:

- Swelling of the face and neck.
- Unexplained weight loss.
- Swelling of glands in head, neck, or armpits.
- Recurring pneumonia or bronchitis.
- Shortness of breath and wheezing.
- Coughing up blood.
- Persistent cough.
- Loss of appetite.
- Fatigue.
- Chest pain.

Showing tumor and bronchoscopic view

Cystic Fibrosis

In cystic fibrosis, a defective gene causes the body to produce an abnormally thick, sticky mucus that clogs the lungs and leads to life-threatening lung infections. These thick secretions also obstruct and may destroy the pancreas, preventing digestive enzymes from reaching the intestines to help with break down and absorption of food.

Signs and Symptoms:

- Persistent cough and mucus production.
- Wheezing and shortness of breath.
- Greasy, bulky stools.
- Salty-tasting skin.
- Poor weight gain.
- Recurrent sinus infections.

Showing thick, sticky mucus

Pneumonia

Pneumonia is an infection in which the air sacs in the lungs become filled with pus or other fluids. This can impair oxygen delivery through the lungs to other tissue and can cause cells to function improperly.

Signs and Symptoms:

- Sputum (*phlegm*) production.
- Chest pain on inspiration (*breathing in*).
- Shaking chills.
- Cough.
- Fever.

Showing inflammation and bacteria

Asthma

Asthma is a disease in which the bronchial airways of the lungs become narrow. An asthma episode is the body's reaction to an irritating substance or allergen that has been inhaled. During an asthma episode, the walls of the airways in the lungs become narrowed, thick, and swollen with sticky mucus, making breathing difficult.

Signs and Symptoms:

- Tightness in the neck and/or chest area.
- Wheezing or coughing, especially at night or after exercise.
- Difficulty breathing.
- Symptoms may worsen during an upper respiratory or sinus infection.

Showing narrowed airway and increased mucus

©2014 Wolters Kluwer

Risks of Obesity

50

What Is Obesity?

Obesity has become a major public health problem, with both genetic and environmental causes. The term *obesity* is simply defined as too much body fat. The percentage of body tissue that is body fat varies according to gender and age. People are considered obese if their weight is 20% or more above their ideal weight range. Morbid obesity is when a people are 50% or more above their ideal weight range. Obesity is a long-term disease that increases the risk of developing other serious health problems, including high blood pressure, high blood cholesterol, Type 2 diabetes, heart disease and stroke.

Causes of Obesity

Obesity usually results from more than one cause. The main cause of obesity is energy imbalance. It is when more energy (calories) is taken from food than is used through physical activity. Weight gain is the result, and the excess energy is stored as fat. Other factors that can contribute to a person's weight are age, gender, genetics, environmental factors, psychological factors, illness and medication.

Treatment for Adult Obesity

Obesity is a chronic disease and it needs long-term management. The focus usually is to reduce the risk for developing health problems, as well as to lose the excess weight. If you are obese, it is best to consult a healthcare professional to help determine how much weight you should lose and what kind of weight loss program is appropriate.

A good plan is to gradually reduce your weight. Weight loss of one to two pounds per week is a safe and healthy strategy. A successful treatment plan can include one or more of the following options: diet, physical activity, behavioral therapy, counseling, drug therapy, and surgery.

Diet

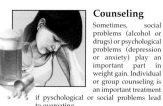

For weight loss, a low calorie, well-balanced diet that is low in fat is recommended. Dietary therapy involves reducing the number of calories that are eaten and learning how to select portion sizes, which types of food to buy, and how to read nutrition labels. Speak with a healthcare professional to determine your ideal calorie intake.

Physical Activity

Daily physical activity is important for weight loss, maintenance of weight loss, and general good health. Physical activity doesn't only involve exercise. It also includes everyday activities such as walking up stairs or yard work. Adults should have at least 30 minutes of moderate physical activity daily.

Counseling

Sometimes, social problems (alcohol or drugs) or psychological problems (depression or anxiety) play an important part in weight gain. Individual or group counseling is an important treatment if pyschological or social problems lead to overeating.

Drug Therapy

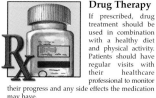

If prescribed, drug treatment should be used in combination with a healthy diet and physical activity. Patients should have regular visits with their healthcare professional to monitor their progress and any side effects the medication may have.

Surgery

Surgery should be considered only for patients with severe obesity who have not been able to lose weight with other treatment options and who are at high risk for developing other life-threatening health problems. The goal of these types of surgeries is to modify the gastrointestinal tract to reduce the amount of food that can be eaten.

Behavioral Therapy

A successful weight loss plan involves changing eating and physical activity habits to new patterns that will promote successful weight loss and weight control.

Behavioral therapy can include strategies such as keeping a food diary to help recognize eating habits; identifying high-risk situations (having high-calorie foods in the house) and then consciously avoiding them; and changing unrealistic beliefs related to a patient's body image. A support network such as family, friends or a support group, is beneficial as well.

How Is Body Fat Measured?

There are two ways in which body fat is measured: **waist circumference** and **body mass index (BMI)**. Waist circumference is a common measurement used to assess abdominal (stomach) fat. People with excess fat that is situated mostly around the abdomen are at risk for many of the serious conditions associated with obesity. A high-risk waistline is one that is 35 inches or greater in women and 40 inches or greater in men.

BMI is a measure of weight in relation to a person's height. For most people, BMI has a strong relationship to weight. To calculate your BMI use the following equations:

English Formula

$$BMI = \left(\frac{\text{weight in pounds}}{\text{(height in inches) x (height in inches)}} \right) \times 703$$

or

Metric Formula

$$BMI = \frac{\text{weight in kilograms}}{\text{(height in meters) x (height in meters)}}$$

Healthy weight: BMI from 18.5 to 25   **Overweight:** BMI from 25 to 30   **Obese:** BMI 30 or greater

For adults, BMI can also be found by using the table below. To use the BMI table, first find your weight at the bottom of the graph. Go straight up from that point until you reach the line that matches your height. Then look to see what weight group you fall in.

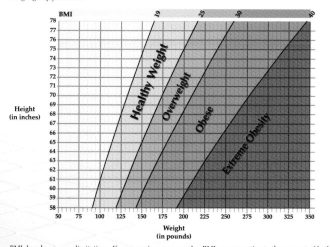

BMI does have some limitations. If a person is very muscular, BMI can overestimate the amount of body fat. It can also underestimate body fat if a person has lost muscle mass, as in the elderly. An actual diagnosis of obesity should be made by a health professional.

Obesity and Children

The prevalence of child obesity is increasing rapidly worldwide. In the U.S. alone, 1 out of 5 children is overweight. When compared to children with a healthy weight, overweight children are more likely to have an increased risk of heart disease, high blood pressure, and Type 2 diabetes. Children who are obese are also more likely to grow up to be obese adults. As with adults, lack of exercise, unhealthy eating habits, genetics and lifestyle all can influence a child's weight.

Doctors or healthcare professionals are the best people to help determine if your child is overweight. By considering your child's age and growth patterns, they can decide if the child's weight is healthy.

Health Risks Associated with Obesity

If you are obese, you have a greater risk of developing serious health problems. If you lose weight, the risk is reduced. The following is a list of diseases and disorders that can develop as a result of obesity.

(A) Brain
Psychological disorders (low-self esteem, depression), stroke

(B) Esophagus
Gastroesophageal reflux disease (GERD), heartburn

(C) Arteries
High blood pressure, arteriosclerosis (atherosclerosis, arteriolar sclerosis), high blood cholesterol

(D) Lungs
Asthma, sleep apnea (interrupted breathing while sleeping)

(E) Heart
Coronary heart disease, heart attack

(F) Gallbladder
Gallstones, cancer, inflammation of the gallbladder, gallbladder disease

(G) Pancreas
Insulin resistance, Type 2 diabetes, hyperinsulinemia

(H) Kidneys
Cancer, uric acid nephrolithiasis (stones in the kidneys)

(I) Colon
Cancer

(J) Bladder
Cancer, bladder control problems (stress incontinence)

(K) Bones
Gout (type of arthritis that deposits uric acid within the joints), osteoarthritis (degeneration of cartilage and bone in the joints)

Other possible health consequences of obesity include endometrial, breast, and prostate cancer; poor female reproductive health (menstrual irregularities, infertility, irregular ovulation, complications of pregnancy) and premature death.

©2014 Wolters Kluwer

How Pain Works

3 Brain processes the message and alerts the body of pain.

Brain

Spinal cord

Nerves

2 Nerves pick up the injury and send the message to the brain.

- *Red dashed line show message flow from pain site to brain.*
- *Blue dotted line show message going from brain to pain site.*

1 Injury occurs in the body.

What Is Pain?

It is an unpleasant sensation occurring in varying degrees of severity associated with injury, disease, or emotional disorder.

2 Types of Pain

1. ACUTE PAIN

occurs as a result of injury to the body and generally disappears when the physical injury heals. Acute pain is linked to tissue injury. Anxiety is common with acute pain.

Examples include:
- Surgical pain
- Muscle strains
- Orthopedic-type injuries
- Labor and delivery

Symptoms: Patient is able to point to site of pain.
- Sharp
- Burning
- Cramping
- Aching
- Pressured

2. CHRONIC (PERSISTENT) PAIN

lasts beyond the normal healing period – usually at least 3 months. The pain may be multifocal and vague. There may be no signs on x-rays or scans to indicate the source of the pain since some pain may be generated by tissue injury. Depression is common with chronic pain.

Neuropathic chronic pain is a type of pain that is caused by injury to a nerve. Patients describe the pain as having tingling, numbness, or burning sensation. Neuropathic pain is difficult to treat.

Common types of neuropathic chronic pain include:
- Diabetic neuropathy – nerve damage as a result of high blood sugar.
- Post-herpetic neuralgia – pain from shingles after the blisters have healed.
- HIV/AIDS – pain from the viral illness or the drugs used to treat the disease.
- Peripheral vascular disease – pain in legs, usually during activity, from lack of blood supply to the extremities. The legs may be discolored, cold, and the skin may be shiny.

Symptoms:
- Painful itching
- Strange sensations
- Extreme sensitivity to normal touch and temperature
- Burning
- Electric-like sensation
- Painful numbness
- Pins and needles

Non-neuropathic chronic pain is pain that is not caused by injury to a nerve.

The most common types include:
- Low back pain – pain in the lower back from muscles, ligaments, tendons, arthritis, or damaged discs.
- Osteoarthritis – arthritis resulting from wear and tear of the joints and with normal aging.
- Rheumatoid arthritis – an autoimmune disorder resulting in pain, stiffness, and inflammation of the joints.

Symptoms: Poorly localized pain (patient may not be able to point to site of pain).
- Gnawing
- Pounding
- Deep aching

Unknown: There are many common chronic pain syndromes that are neither known to be chronic non-neuropathic nor neuropathic.

These include:
- Fibromyalgia syndrome – diffuse body pain with tenderness in the muscles.
- Tension headache – pressure-type headache lasting days to weeks and often not severe.
- Migraine headache – episodic headache that persists for hours to days with nausea and is often severe.
- Irritable bowel syndrome (IBS) – abdominal pain with cramping, bloating, and constipation often alternating with diarrhea.
- Some low back pain – back pain that is not muscular, not related to disc injury, and without a known cause.

Symptoms: May be a combination of chronic non-neuropathic and neuropathic symptoms.

Treatment

Specific treatment options need to be tailored to the individual patient. Be sure to consult with your healthcare professional to determine the right treatment for you.

Prevention techniques:
- Regular exercise   • Maintain a healthy body weight   • Use safe techniques when lifting heavy objects

Right   Left

Where do you Feel Pain?

Left   Right

Pain Scale

0 1 2 3 4 5 6 7 8 9 10

No pain   *Rate your pain by choosing the number that best describes it.*   *Extreme pain*

©2014 Wolters Kluwer

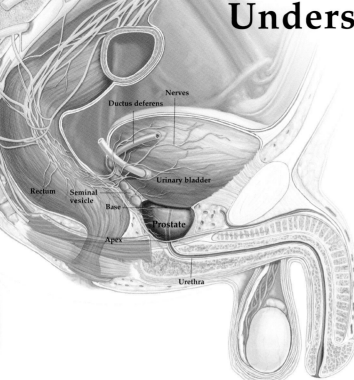

What is Prostate Cancer?

Prostate cancer is cancer of the walnut-sized gland of a man's reproductive system that makes part of the seminal fluid, which carries sperm out of the body.

Risk Factors

The causes of prostate cancer are not known. Below are some factors, which research has shown could increase a man's risk of developing prostate cancer.

Age - The primary risk of prostate cancer increases with age.

Family history - The risk of prostate cancer increases if a close male family member (father or brother) has had the disease.

Race or ethnicity - African American men are more likely to develop prostate cancer.

Geographic location - There is a higher incidence of prostate cancer in men residing in North America, Northwest Europe, and Australia, in part due to pre-screening. There is a lower incidence in men residing in Asia and in some developing countries.

Diet - A diet high in fat and red meat may increase a man's risk of developing prostate cancer. Although the data is limited, eating cruciferous vegetables (such as broccoli), tomatoes and soybeans may decrease the risk of this disease.

Staging and Gleason Score

To plan treatment, the physician must understand the extent (stage) and how fast the cancer will grow and spread (which is best determined by the Gleason score).

Gleason Score - The system of grading the aggressiveness of the cancer is the Gleason Pathologic Scoring System, which scores or grades the cancer from 1 to 5. To get a Gleason score, the two most common areas of cancer are scored individually and added together for a Gleason score between 2 and 10. A lower score indicates a less aggressive cancer and a higher score indicates a more aggressive cancer.

Gleason Pathologic Scoring System

How your cells look under a microscope determines the Gleason score. Based on appearance, the pathologist can identify which cells are normal, which are cancer cells and how aggressive those cells are.

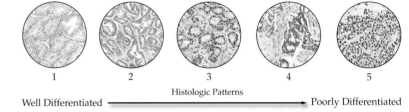

1   2   3   4   5

Histologic Patterns

Well Differentiated ⟶ Poorly Differentiated

Staging - The cancer stage is based on the size and spread of the tumor; the higher the stage, the more advanced the cancer. The most commonly used system is the Tumor- Nodes- Metastasis system (TNM).

T = the size and location of the primary **Tumor**

N = the number of lymph **Nodes** to which the cancer has spread

M = the spread away from the primary site of the tumor to other parts of the body is **Metastasis**

Signs & Symptoms

Many men with prostate cancer do not experience any symptoms when they are diagnosed. While the symptoms listed below may be due to prostate cancer, they can also be associated with other non-cancerous conditions.

• **Erection difficulties**
• **Blood in semen**
• **Pain in lower back, hips, upper thighs**
• **Urinary problems,** which can include:
 - Difficulties starting or stopping the flow of urine
 - Urine flow that starts and stops
 - Needing to urinate often, especially at night
 - Weak urine flow
 - Pain or burning sensation during urination
 - Blood in the urine

Screening and Diagnosis

Screening can help find and treat cancer early. Men may want to see their doctor to discuss prostate cancer screening if they are over the age of 50, have any of the risk factors, or are experiencing any of the symptoms. Some common screening tests include:

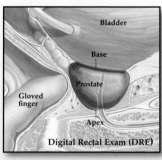

Digital Rectal Exam (DRE)

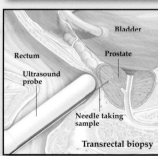

Transrectal biopsy

Blood test for Prostate-Specific Antigen (PSA) - PSA is a substance produced by the prostate that helps keep semen liquid. A blood test is performed to test the level of PSA. Although high levels of PSA could indicate cancer, other causes could include inflammation of the prostate or Benign Prostatic Hyperplasia (BPH).

Digital rectal exam (DRE) - Most tumors arise in the area of the prostate (peripheral zone) which can be detected by the DRE.

Depending on the results of the screening test(s), the physician will perform additional diagnostic tests, which may include:

Transrectal ultrasound - A probe inserted into a man's rectum can better determine the exact size and location of the abnormal areas.

Transrectal biopsy - By inserting a needle through the rectum into the prostate, tissue is removed to look for cancer cells.

Endorectal MRI – A probe inserted into a man's rectum can obtain sharp images of the prostate and identify suspicious areas.

Other imaging tests such as a bone scan, CT scan or MRI may be performed to determine if the cancer has spread to other parts of the body.

Treatments

There are several ways to treat prostate cancer and a combination of treatments may be recommended by the physician. Treatment will depend on a number of factors such as the PSA level, the Gleason score (indicates how aggressive the cancer is), spread (stage) of the cancer, as well as the age, symptoms, and health of the patient.

Common treatment options include:

Surgery - The procedure can include removal of all or part of the prostate gland.

Radiation therapy - Radiation treatment can be external, which uses a high-powered X-ray machine outside the body to kill cancer cells. Radiation can also be internal, by implanting small radioactive "seeds" inside the prostate tissue.

Hormone therapy -Medication is used to stop or block the production of male sex hormones which stimulate the growth of cancer cells.

Active surveillance or "Watchful waiting" (because prostate cancer can be very slow growing) - If the risks or possible side effects of the treatment options above outweigh the benefits, the physician may recommend close monitoring of the cancer to determine growth rate. If disease characteristics get worse or symptoms occur, then the above treatment options may be considered.

Prognostic factors

Like other forms of cancer, the prognosis for prostate cancer stage depends on how far the cancer has spread at the time it's diagnosed. Gleason score, PSA, Stage and volume of disease (determined by biopsy information) are the main factors that affect the outcome. Talk to your cancer specialist if you are trying to find out about your prognosis.

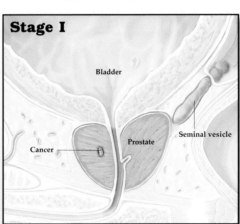

Stage I

The cancer is not found during a digital rectal exam (T1), but found when doing a biopsy for increased PSA or surgery for another reason. It is located only in the prostate.

T1, N0, M0, PSA<10, Gleason ≤6

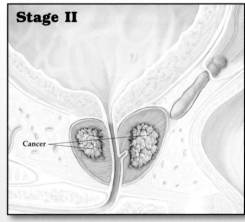

Stage II

The tumor is not felt on the digital rectal exam (T1) but the PSA or Gleason score is higher than stage 1, or the tumor can be felt but is confined to the gland.

Stage IIA : T1, N0, M0, PSA 10-20, Gleason 6
 OR   T1, N0, M0, PSA<20, Gleason 7
 OR   T2a-b (tumor felt on one side only) N0, M0, PSA<20, Gleason ≤7

Stage IIB : T1-2, N0, M0, PSA≤20 and/or Gleason≤8
 OR   T2c (tumor felt on both sides) N0, M0

Stage III

The cancer has spread outside the prostate, perhaps to the seminal vesicles, but not to the lymph nodes

T3, N0, M0, any PSA, any Gleason

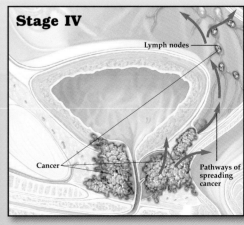

Stage IV

The cancer may have spread to nearby muscles, organs, lymph nodes or other parts of the body.

T4, N1, M1, any PSA, any Gleason

©2014 Wolters Kluwer

53

Sexually Transmitted Infections

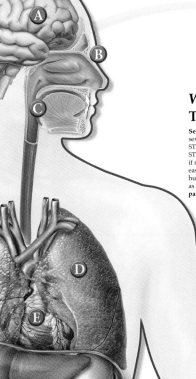

What Are Sexually Transmitted Infections?

Sexually transmitted infections (STIs) are diseases you can get by having sex with someone who has an infection. There are more than 20 types of STIs, which can be spread during vaginal, oral, and anal sexual contact. STIs can be painful, and may have serious consequences (including death) if not treated. **Bacterial** STIs like gonorrhea and chlamydia are relatively easy to cure if treated early, but **viral** STIs, like genital herpes and the human immunodeficiency virus (HIV) cannot be cured. Other STIs such as trichomoniasis are caused by **protozoa** (single-celled organisms), and **parasites** are responsible for pubic lice and scabies.

Complications

Without treatment, sexually transmitted infections can lead to serious health problems— especially in women. In addition, STIs increase the risk of acquiring and transmitting HIV, the virus that causes AIDS. Some complications of STIs and the organs affected are listed below:

(A) Brain and Nervous System - Headaches, brain damage, meningitis (inflamed lining of the brain), stroke, neurological disorders (nervous system problems), psychiatric illness, spinal damage

(B) Eyes - Conjunctivitis, blindness

(C) Mouth and Throat - Thrush (infection of the oral tissues), pharyngitis (inflamed throat)

(D) Lungs - Peumocystis carinii (form of pneumonia common in people with reduced immunity)

(E) Heart and Blood Vessels - Aortic stenosis (narrowing of artery and/or valve of the heart), inflammation of the aorta, aneurysm (bulging) of the aorta, Kaposi's sarcoma (AIDS-related cancer affecting walls of certain lymphatic vessels)

(F) Skin - Rashes, itching, blisters, ulcers

(G) Intestines - Dysentery (inflammation of the intestine, with abdominal pain and frequent, watery stools)

(H) Urinary System - Cystitis (inflammation of the bladder), urinary tract infections, urethritis (inflammation of urethra)

(I) Bones and Joints - Arthritis, bone aches

Reproductive system complications include:

Male– Prostatitis (inflammation of the prostate gland), sterility, impotence, epididymitis (inflammation of the epididymis), urethral stricture

Female– Pelvic scarring, genital damage, cervical cancer, infertility, vulvovaginitis (inflammation of vulva and vagina), ectopic (tubal) pregnancy

Signs and Symptoms

The table below lists some of the most common symptoms of STIs. It is important to remember that many women and men who have an STI often do not experience any symptoms at all. If you are experiencing any of the symptoms listed below or if you believe you have an STI, talk to your health care provider as soon as possible.

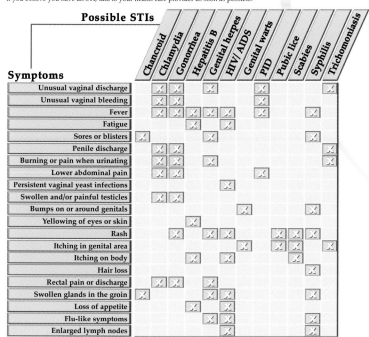

Possible STIs

Symptoms	Chancroid	Chlamydia	Gonorrhea	Hepatitis B	Genital herpes	HIV/AIDS	Genital warts	PID	Pubic lice	Scabies	Syphilis	Trichomoniasis
Unusual vaginal discharge		X	X					X				X
Unusual vaginal bleeding		X	X					X				
Fever		X	X	X	X	X		X			X	
Fatigue				X		X						
Sores or blisters	X				X						X	
Penile discharge		X	X									X
Burning or pain when urinating		X	X		X							X
Lower abdominal pain		X	X					X				
Persistent vaginal yeast infections						X						
Swollen and/or painful testicles		X	X									
Bumps on or around genitals							X			X		
Yellowing of eyes or skin				X								
Rash				X	X	X				X	X	
Itching in genital area					X				X	X		X
Itching on body				X		X				X		
Hair loss											X	
Rectal pain or discharge		X	X		X							
Swollen glands in the groin	X				X	X					X	
Loss of appetite				X		X						
Flu-like symptoms					X	X					X	
Enlarged lymph nodes						X					X	

Genital Warts

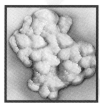

Genital warts are painless growths found on or around the genital and anal areas. They are caused by the human papillomavirus (HPV). Despite treatment, genital warts cannot be cured and often recur. In women, infection with certain strains of HPV can increase the risk of developing cervical cancer.

Genital Herpes

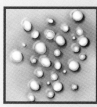

Genital herpes is a viral infection that causes painful sores on and around the genitals or anal area. It is easily spread and the disease tends to recur, especially in the first few years after initial infection. There is no cure, but there are medications that can help relieve symptoms.

Chancroid

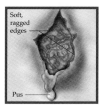

Soft, ragged edges / Pus

Chancroid (shan-kroid) is a bacterial infection that causes painful ulcers on the genitals. The chancroid ulcer can be difficult to distinguish from ulcers that are caused by genital herpes and syphilis. Symptoms usually appear within a week of exposure.

Syphilis

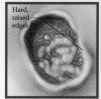

Hard, raised edges

Syphilis is a bacterial infection, that can damage organs over time if untreated. The first symptom of syphilis is an ulcer called a **chancre** (shan-ker). Left untreated, about one-third of cases will go onto the later, more damaging, stages.

Trichomoniasis

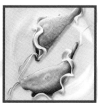

One of the most common STIs, trichomoniasis (trick-oh-moh-nye-uh-sis) is a genital-tract infection caused by a protozoan (single-celled organism). This STI is usually transmitted through sexual intercourse, but a woman can also transmit the infection to her baby during childbirth.

HIV/AIDS

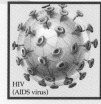

HIV (AIDS virus)

HIV (human immuno-deficiency virus) infects and gradually destroys cells in the immune system. HIV severely weakens the body's response to infections and cancers. Eventually, AIDS (acquired immunodeficiency syndrome) is diagnosed. With AIDS, a variety of infections can overtake the body and eventually cause death.

Pelvic Inflammatory Disease (PID)

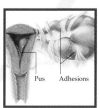

Pus   Adhesions

PID is a term used to describe an infection of the uterus, fallopian tubes or ovaries. It is the most common, serious infection among young women. PID infection can cause scarring of the tissue inside the fallopian tubes, which can damage the tubes or block them completely. If untreated, PID can result in infertility, ectopic pregnancy, miscarriage, or chronic pain.

Hepatitis B

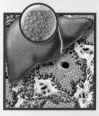

The liver disease Hepatitis B is caused by a virus carried in the blood, saliva, semen, and other body fluids of an infected person. It is spread through sexual contact and can be spread from a mother to her baby during childbirth or during breastfeeding. Recovery usually happens within six months, but in rare cases hepatitis B can lead to liver damage and an increased risk of liver cancer.

Pubic Lice

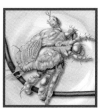

Pubic lice are tiny parasites that live in pubic hair and survive by feeding on human blood. They are most often spread by sexual activity, but in rare cases they can be spread through contact with infested clothing or bedding. It is unusual for pubic lice to cause any serious health problems, but the itching they cause can be very uncomfortable.

Scabies

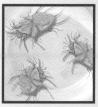

Scabies is a parasitic skin infection caused by a tiny mite. Highly contagious, it is spread primarily through sexual contact, though it also can be spread through contact with skin, infested clothing, or bedding. Scabies causes intense itching, which often is worse at night.

Chlamydia

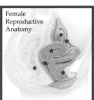

Female Reproductive Anatomy

Chlamydia is a bacterial infection very similar to gonorrhea. Up to 50 percent of men, and 75 percent of women don't experience any symptoms. Complications for women are more serious than for men. In women chlamydia can cause irreversible damage, such as pelvic inflammatory disease and infertility.

★ = sites of chlamydia and gonorrhea infection

Gonorrhea

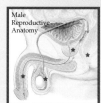

Male Reproductive Anatomy

Gonorrhea, is a curable STI which can infect the genital tract, the mouth, and the rectum. It is usually spread through sexual contact, but an infected woman can pass the disease to her baby during delivery. Often there are no symptoms. Untreated it can cause sterility in both sexes.

★ = sites of chlamydia and gonorrhea infection

Prevention and Treatment

The only way to eliminate the risk of acquiring an STI is to avoid sex *completely*. But there are several measures you can take to *reduce* your risk and to avoid transmitting STIs:

- Avoid sex with multiple partners.
- Use a condom.
- Get a Hepatitis B immunization (shot).
- Become familiar with the symptoms of STIs.
- Know your sexual partner's sexual history.
- Have regular checkups for STIs, even if you have no symptoms.
- Seek medical help immediately if any suspicious symptoms develop.
- If infected, tell any past or present partner(s) so that they may get treated.
- Avoid all sexual activity while being treated for an STI.

Most STIs are easily treated. The earlier a person seeks treatment, the less likely the disease will cause permanent physical damage, be spread to others, or be passed on from a mother to her newborn baby.

©2014 Wolters Kluwer

54

Dangers of Smoking

Tobacco smoke is a highly dangerous substance that contains more than 200 known poisons. Every time a smoker lights up, he or she is being injured to some degree by inhaling these poisons. A two-pack-a-day smoker shortens his or her life expectancy by eight years, and even light smokers shorten their life expectancy by four years. To date, lung cancer is the leading cause of death in men, yet incidence is increasing among women often resulting in death at an earlier age than men.

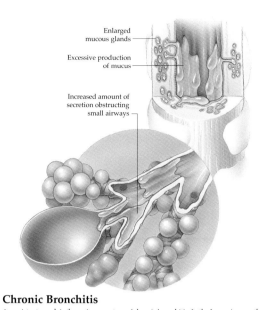

Enlarged mucous glands

Excessive production of mucus

Increased amount of secretion obstructing small airways

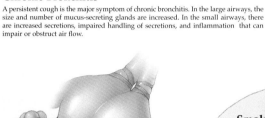

Chronic Bronchitis

A persistent cough is the major symptom of chronic bronchitis. In the large airways, the size and number of mucus-secreting glands are increased. In the small airways, there are increased secretions, impaired handling of secretions, and inflammation that can impair or obstruct air flow.

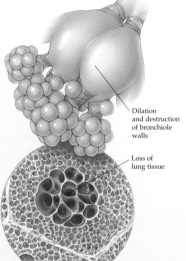

Dilation and destruction of bronchiole walls

Loss of lung tissue

Emphysema

With emphysema, the lungs irreversibly lose their ability to take up oxygen, causing great breathing difficulty. Lung tissue loses its elasticity, air sacs tear, and stale air becomes trapped, eventually causing death from lack of oxygen.

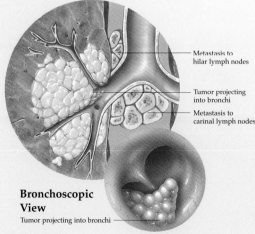

Metastasis to hilar lymph nodes

Tumor projecting into bronchi

Metastasis to carinal lymph nodes

Bronchoscopic View

Tumor projecting into bronchi

Lung Cancer

Tobacco smoke is the most common cause of lung cancer. One in ten heavy smokers will get lung cancer, and in most cases it will be fatal. It is the leading cause of death by cancer because it is difficult to detect, and it is likely to spread early to the liver, brain, and bones.

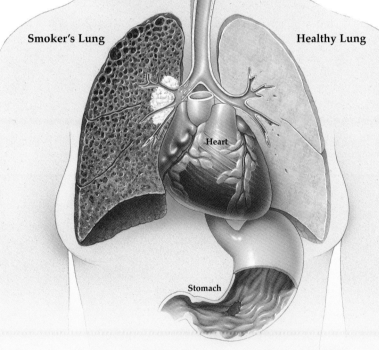

Brain

Tongue

Smoker's Lung

Healthy Lung

Heart

Stomach

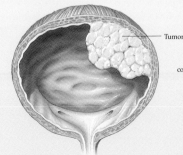

Tumor

Bladder Cancer

Chemicals from tobacco are absorbed into the bloodstream and leave the body through the urine. These cancer-causing chemicals are always in contact with the bladder, increasing the risk for bladder cancer.

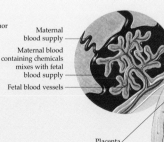

Maternal blood supply

Maternal blood containing chemicals mixes with fetal blood supply

Fetal blood vessels

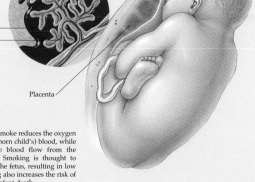

Placenta

Fetal Risk

Carbon monoxide in smoke reduces the oxygen level in the fetus' (unborn child's) blood, while nicotine restricts the blood flow from the mother to the fetus. Smoking is thought to retard the growth of the fetus, resulting in low birth weight. Smoking also increases the risk of premature birth and infant death.

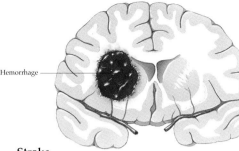

Hemorrhage

Stroke

Smoking is a major cause of arteriosclerosis, or hardening of the arteries. In turn, arteriosclerosis is a chief cause of stroke. Strokes occur when one of the arteries of the brain ruptures, forms a blood clot, or bleeds into the brain. Once brain tissue is destroyed it cannot be repaired.

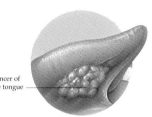

Mouth and Throat Cancer

Cancer-causing chemicals from tobacco products increase the risk of cancer of the lip, cheek, tongue, and larynx (voice box). The removal of these cancers can be disfiguring and can result in loss of the larynx.

Cancer of the tongue

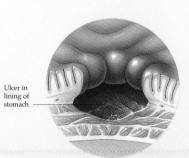

Plaque in coronary artery wall

Heart Disease

Arteriosclerosis is responsible for most heart attacks. Plaque, deposits of cholesterol, collecting in the coronary arteries narrows the vessels until eventually the oxygen supply to the heart is stopped. Smoking accelerates this process.

Ulcer in lining of stomach

Gastric Ulcer

Smoking increases the production of gastric juices, raising the acidity level and eroding the lining of the stomach. Painful ulcers result from these eroded areas and increase the risk for hemorrhage and perforation of the stomach lining.

©2014 Wolters Kluwer

Human Spine Disorders

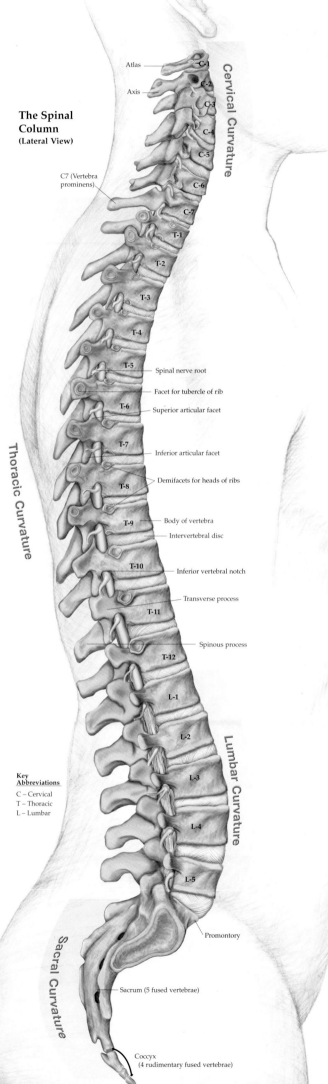

55

The Spinal Column
(Lateral View)

Atlas
Axis
C-1
C-2
C-3
C-4
C-5
C-6
C-7
C7 (Vertebra prominens)
Cervical Curvature

T-1
T-2
T-3
T-4
T-5 — Spinal nerve root
T-6 — Facet for tubercle of rib
— Superior articular facet
T-7 — Inferior articular facet
T-8 — Demifacets for heads of ribs
T-9 — Body of vertebra
— Intervertebral disc
T-10 — Inferior vertebral notch
— Transverse process
T-11
— Spinous process
T-12
Thoracic Curvature

L-1
L-2
L-3
L-4
L-5
Lumbar Curvature
Promontory

Key Abbreviations
C – Cervical
T – Thoracic
L – Lumbar

Sacrum (5 fused vertebrae)
Sacral Curvature

Coccyx
(4 rudimentary fused vertebrae)

Anatomy

A Typical Cervical Vertebra (Superior View)

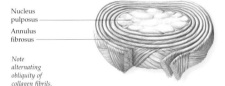

Spinous process
Internal vertebral venous plexus
Dura mater
Lamina
Arachnoid mater
Spinal cord
Pia mater
Dorsal root of spinal nerve
Superior articular facet
Ventral root of spinal nerve
Root sheath
Spinal ganglion
Vertebral veins
Posterior longitudinal ligament
Vertebral artery
Pedicle
Annulus fibrosus
Vertebral body
Intervertebral cartilage (disc)
Nucleus pulposus
Anterior longitudinal ligament

Typical Vertebrae (Superior View)

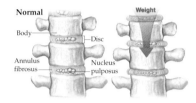

Cervical vertebra
Thoracic vertebra
Lumbar vertebra

Structural Features of an Intervertebral Disc (Schematic)

Nucleus pulposus
Annulus fibrosus

Note alternating obliquity of collagen fibrils.

The nucleus pulposus is the central gelatinous cushioning part of the intervertebral disc enclosed in several layers of cartilaginous laminae. The nucleus pulposus becomes dehydrated with age.

Function of Intervertebral Discs

Normal
Weight
Body
Disc
Annulus fibrosus
Nucleus pulposus

The disc, which contains nucleus pulposus, functions to protect the vertebrae from pressure.

Pathology

Osteoporosis

Osteoporosis develops when the body loses bone more quickly than it can make new bone. As a result, bones become less dense at the core and lose thickness at the surface. This increases the bones' susceptibility to fracture.

When osteoporosis involves the lumbar region, the vertebral bodies become markedly biconcave and the discs are ballooned.

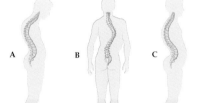

Compression fractures commonly occur at the thoracolumbar vertebral junction, resulting in wedge-shaped vertebrae.

* Fractures of laminae, pedicles, or transverse processes of the vertebrae are common.

A   B   C

A. Hyperkyphosis
An excessive rounding of the thoracic vertebral column (humpback or hunchback).

B. Scoliosis
A curvature of the spine, often with twisting of the spinal column.

C. Hyperlordosis
A forward/anterior curvature of the cervical and lumbar (lower back) regions of the spine. In the lumbar region, it is also called "swayback."

Causes of Pain in the Back or Extremities

Shown below are other causes of pain that the examining physician should consider in making the diagnosis.

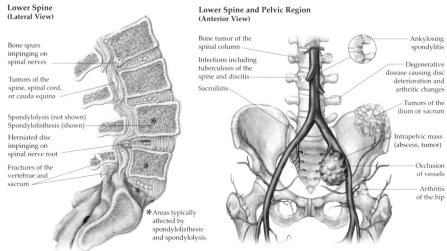

Lower Spine (Lateral View)

Bone spurs impinging on spinal nerves
Tumors of the spine, spinal cord, or cauda equina
Spondylolysis (not shown)
Spondylolisthesis (shown)
Herniated disc impinging on spinal nerve root
Fractures of the vertebrae and sacrum

* Areas typically affected by spondylolisthesis and spondylolysis.

Lower Spine and Pelvic Region (Anterior View)

Bone tumor of the spinal column
Infections including tuberculosis of the spine and discitis
Sacroiliitis
Ankylosing spondylitis
Degenerative disease causing disc deterioration and arthritic changes
Tumors of the ilium or sacrum
Intrapelvic mass (abscess, tumor)
Occlusion of vessels
Arthritis of the hip

©2014 Wolters Kluwer

56

Understanding Stroke

What Is Stroke?

Stroke refers to the sudden death of brain tissue caused by a lack of oxygen resulting from an interrupted blood supply. An **infarct** is the area of the brain that has "died" because of this lack of oxygen. There are two ways that brain tissue death can occur. **Ischemic stroke** is a blockage or reduction of blood flow in an artery that feeds that area of the brain. It is the most common cause of an infarct. **Hemorrhagic stroke** results from bleeding within and around the brain causing compression and tissue injury.

Ischemic Stroke

This type of stroke results from a blockage or reduction of blood flow to an area of the brain. This blockage may result from atherosclerosis and blood clot formation.

Atherosclerosis is the deposit of cholesterol and plaque within the walls of arteries. These deposits may become large enough to narrow the lumen and reduce the flow of blood while also causing the artery to lose its ability to stretch.

A **thrombus**, or blood clot, forms on the roughened surface of atherosclerotic plaques that develop in the wall of the artery. The thrombus can enlarge and eventually block the lumen of the artery.

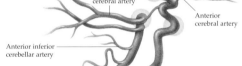

- Lumen
- Plaque
- Thrombus

Common Sites of Plaque Formation
(Indicated by yellow circles)

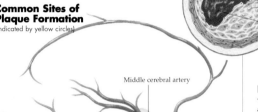

- Middle cerebral artery
- Posterior cerebral artery
- Anterior cerebral artery
- Anterior inferior cerebellar artery
- Posterior inferior cerebellar artery
- Embolus
- Internal carotid artery
- Embolus
- Vertebral artery
- Common carotid artery

Part of a thrombus may break off and become an **embolus**. An embolus travels through the blood stream until it reaches a vessel too small for it to pass through, thus blocking it.

Emboli commonly come from the heart, where different diseases can cause thrombus formation.

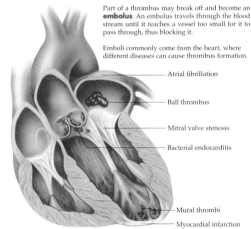

- Atrial fibrillation
- Ball thrombus
- Mitral valve stenosis
- Bacterial endocarditis
- Mural thrombi
- Myocardial infarction

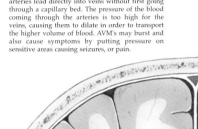

- Intracerebral hemorrhage
- Arteriovenous malformation (AVM)

Hemorrhagic Stroke

This type of stroke is caused by bleeding within and around the brain. Bleeding that fills the spaces between the brain and the skull is called a **subarachnoid hemorrhage**. It is caused by ruptured aneurysms, arteriovenous malformations, and head trauma. Bleeding within the brain tissue itself is known as **intracerebral hemorrhage** and is primarily caused by hypertension.

An **aneurysm** is a weakening of the arterial wall that causes it to stretch and balloon. It usually occurs where the artery branches.

Hypertension is an elevation of blood pressure that may cause tiny arterioles to burst causing the tissue beyond the rupture to die. Blood vessels in the dead tissue then leak causing more bleeding.

- Circle of Willis
- Aneurysm

An **arteriovenous malformation** (AVM) is an abnormality of the brain's blood vessels in which arteries lead directly into veins without first going through a capillary bed. The pressure of the blood coming through the arteries is too high for the veins, causing them to dilate in order to transport the higher volume of blood. AVM's may burst and also cause symptoms by putting pressure on sensitive areas causing seizures, or pain.

- Microaneurysm
- Arterioles
- Subarachnoid hemorrhage

Normal Functional Areas of Brain

The brain has two sides: a right hemisphere that controls the left side of the body and a left hemisphere that controls the right side of the body. Each hemisphere has four lobes and a cerebellum that control our daily functions. Depending on what part of the brain has been affected, stroke victims experience a variety of neurological deficits. Rehabilitation is crucial to the stroke patient's recovery. Physical therapists and speech therapists help patients "relearn" their lost functions and devise ways to cope with the loss of those they cannot regain.

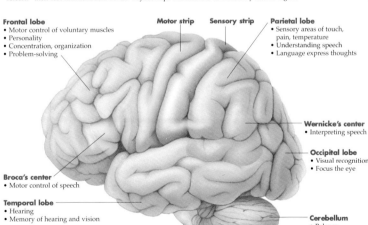

Frontal lobe
- Motor control of voluntary muscles
- Personality
- Concentration, organization
- Problem-solving

Motor strip **Sensory strip**

Parietal lobe
- Sensory areas of touch, pain, temperature
- Understanding speech
- Language express thoughts

Wernicke's center
- Interpreting speech

Occipital lobe
- Visual recognition
- Focus the eye

Broca's center
- Motor control of speech

Temporal lobe
- Hearing
- Memory of hearing and vision

Cerebellum
- Balance
- Coordinating muscle movement

Brain stem
- Controls heart rate and rate of breathing

Events Leading to Stroke

Stroke victims often have small strokes or "warning signs," before a large permanent attack.

Transient Ischemic Attacks (TIAs) are brief attacks that last anywhere from a few minutes to 24 hours. The symptoms resolve completely and the person returns to normal. It is possible to have several TIAs before a large attack.

Complete Infarction (CI) is an attack that leaves permanent tissue death and results in serious neurological deficits. Recovery is usually not total and takes longer than three weeks.

Common Neurological Deficits After Stroke

Left-sided stroke
- Right-sided paralysis
- Speech/language deficits
- Slow, cautious behavior
- Hemianopsia of right visual field
- Memory loss in language
- Right-sided dysarthria
- Aphasia
- Apraxia

Right-sided stroke
- Left-sided paralysis
- Spatial/perceptual deficits
- Quick, impulsive behavior
- Hemianopsia of left visual field
- Memory loss in performance
- Left-sided dysarthria

Related Terms

Paralysis - Loss of muscle function and sensation

Hemiparesis - Weakness of muscles on one side of body

Hemianopsia - Loss of sight in half of visual field

Aphasia - Difficulty with oral communication, reduced ability to read or write

Apraxia - Apraxia is an inability to perform certain learned purposeful movements (not the result of motor or sensory problems)

Ataxia - Loss of coordinated voluntary movements

Dysarthria - Slurring of speech and "mouth droop" on one side of face due to muscle weakness

Risks for Stroke

Hypertension
Heart disease
Atherosclerosis
Previous TIAs
High cholesterol
High alcohol consumption
Obesity
Diabetes
Bruit noise in carotid artery
Cigarette smoking
Oral contraceptive use
Family history of stroke

©2014 Wolters Kluwer